Health Informatics
(formerly Computers in Health Care)

Kathryn J. Hannah   Marion J. Ball
Series Editors

Health Informatics Series
(formerly Computers in Health Care)

Series Editors
Kathryn J. Hannah   Marion J. Ball

Clinical Decision Support Systems
Theory and Practice
Eta S. Bernet

Dental Informatics
Integrating Technology into the Dental Environment
L.M. Abbey and J. Zimmerman

Health Informatics Series
Evaluating the Organizational Itnpact of Healthcare Information Systems, Second Edition
J.G. Anderson and C.E. Aydin

Ethics and Information Technology
A Case-Based Approach to a Health Care System in Transition
J.G. Anderson and K.W. Goodman

Aspects of the Computer-Based Patient Record
M.J. Ball and M.F. Collen

Performance Improvement Through Information Management
Health Care's Bridge to Success
M.J. Ball and J.V. Douglas

Strategies and Technologies for Healthcare Information
Theory into Practice
M.J. Ball, J.V. Douglas, and D.E. Garets

Nursing Informatics
Where Caring and Technology Meet, Third Edition
M.J. Ball, K.J. Hannah, S.K. Newbold, and J.V. Douglas

Healthcare Information Management Systems
A Practical Guide, Second Edition
M.J. Ball, D.W. Simborg, J.W. Albright, and J.V. Douglas

Healthcare Information Management Systems
Cases, Strategies, and Solutions, Third Edition
M.J. Ball, C.A. Weaver, and J.M. Kiel

Clinical Decision Support Systems
Theory and Practice
E.S. Berner

Strategy and Architecture of Health Care Information Systems
M.K. Bourke

Information Networks for Community Health
P.F. Brennan, S.J. Schneider, and E. Tornquist

Informatics for the Clinical Laboratory
A Practical Guide for the Pathologist
D.F. Cowan

Introduction to Clinical Informatics
P. Degoulet and M. Fieschi

Susan M. Houston   Lisa Anne Bove

Project Management
for Healthcare Informatics

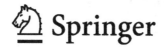 Springer

Susan M. Houston, MBA, RN-BC, PMP
Department of Clinical Research
   Informatics
National Institutes of Health
Bethesda, MD 20892
USA

Lisa Anne Bove, MSN, RN-BC
Management Consultant
Accenture, LLC
Philadelphia, PA 19008
USA

Series Editors:
Kathryn J. Hannah, PhD, RN
Adjunct Professor
Department of Community
   Health Science
Faculty of Medicine
The University of Calgary
Calgary, Alberta T2N 4N1
Canada

Marion J. Ball, EdD
Professor, Johns Hopkins School of Nursing
Joint Appointment
Health Sciences Informatics
Johns Hopkins University School of Nursing
and
Affiliate Professor
Information Systems
University of Maryland
Baltimore
and
Fellow
Global Leadership Initiative
Center for Healthcare Management
Baltimore, MD 21210
USA

ISBN-13: 978-1-4419-2527-5   e-ISBN-13: 978-0-387-73683-9

Printed on acid-free paper.

9 8 7 6 5 4 3 2 1

springer.com

Foreword

The healthcare environment of this millennium is characterized by an unprecedented amount of escalating complexity, pulsating chaos, new technologies, and discontinuous change. There are demands for increased efficiency and effectiveness, with the accompanying constraints of diminishing resources. This presents daily challenges to those committed to creating responsive organizations and positive health outcomes. The need to impose order is being challenged by the assertion that chaos and order are bonded together inseparably. These are like two sides of a coin that form a whole, and both are needed. Healthcare environments, then, are not static machines subject to our control or reducible to their ordered parts. And the work, tasks, or projects that need to be accomplished and managed require more than a walk through sequential steps.

Project management is seen as an important means to navigate through the turbulent environment of the healthcare delivery system to accomplish work, facilitate change, and create improvements. Skill in the project management process then, needs to be developed within the context of a new worldview of organizations, management, and change. The new worldview recognizes that the quintessential act of organizational change is the act of changing our thinking. The skilled project manager is challenged to find the critical path through a series of planned interconnected tasks that can lead to the creation of a new reality. The systematic application of knowledge, skills, tools, and techniques used in the management of projects provides a powerful means to facilitate this change. It is the thoughtful journey through each phase of the project management process that orchestrates different things happening at different times, in different quantities, and at different rates. What appears as chaos on the surface evolves into a new kind of order when project management is done at its best. This is the power and the value of good project management and a good project manager.

Project management is a means of planning for the future. And yet because one cannot predict the future, the project manager needs to be flexible and prepared to alter plans and change course as organizations evolve and the unexpected unfolds. Managing a project is also about managing the participation of others, engaging the talents of many, and mobilizing people around the construction of change. Opening communication, building coalitions, and focusing on action-oriented strategies are all powerful skills that the project manager needs to master. These leadership skills, coupled with an understanding of the project management process, tools, and techniques shared by the authors of this book, will empower both the novice and the veteran project manager. Good project management allows us to walk into chaos, create meaning and order out of complexity, and guide our steps into the future. Effective project managers and successful project management can create a future where the health and safety of the nation are advanced.

Carol A. Romano, PhD, RN, FAAN
Assistant Surgeon General
Chief Nurse Officer US Public Health Service
Senior Advisor for Clinical Research Informatics
Department of Clinical Research Informatics
Clinical Center, National Institutes of Health
May 2007

Series Preface

This series is directed to healthcare professionals who are leading the transformation of health care by using information and knowledge. Launched in 1988 as *Computers in Health Care,* the series offers a broad range of titles: some addressed to specific professions such as nursing, medicine, and health administrations; others to sepcial areas of practice such as trauma and radiology. Still others books in the series focus on interdisciplinary issues, such as the computer-based patient record, electronic health records, and networked healthcare systems

Renamed *Health Informatics* in 1998 to reflect the rapid evolution in the discipline now known as health informatics, the series will continue to add titles that contribute to the evolution of the field. In the series, eminent experts, serving as editors or authors, offer their acounts of innovations in health informatics. Increasingly, these accounts go beyond hardware and software to address the role of information in influencing the transformation of healthcare delivery systems around the world. The series will increasingly focus on "peopleware" and organizational, behavioral, and societal changes that accompany the diffusion of information technology in health services environments.

These changes will shape health services in the new millennium. By making full and creative use of the technology to tame data and to transform information, health informatics will foster the development of the knowledge age in health care. As coeditors, we pledge to support our professional colleagues and the series readers as they share advances in the emerging and exciting field of health informatics.

Kathryn J. Hannah, PhD, RN
Marion J. Ball, EdD

Preface

Project management is defined as "the application of knowledge, skills, tools and techniques to activities to meet project requirements" (PMBOK 2000). Healthcare informatics staff are constantly involved with projects, whether as an analyst defining requirements for a system upgrade, a manager determining projected staffing patterns, a physician championing a new computerized physician order entry system, a staff development instructor creating a critical care course, or an informatics nurse implementing software applications. Knowledge and use of the project management process can assist all levels of healthcare informaticists with all of these projects.

This book will provide a detailed explanation of the project management process using real healthcare examples. Details of each phase of the process, as well as the tools used during each phase, will make up the early chapters of the book. The project management process that is defined as initiation, planning, execution, control, and closing will be described in detail in Chapter 1. Each project management process will be described in detail using templates to demonstrate the work tools and concepts. The following chapters will be devoted to discussion on how to apply these principles in the day-to-day work of the nurse, whether the reader is a manager, staff nurse, educator, researcher, or informaticist.

The initiation phase will be discussed in detail in Chapter 2. The initiation phase authorizes the project to be completed. This chapter will outline the tasks and outcomes to be accomplished during this phase of the project life cycle. The project needs, objectives, and high-level resources are defined. This phase is where the project manager's authority and responsibility are defined. Historical documentation from any previous projects that were similar is useful here and throughout the project. The output of the initiation phase is a project charter or scope document, depending on the size of the project.

Chapter 3 will describe the planning phase. The planning phase selects the best course of action to accomplish the objectives and goals of the project. This chapter will outline that tasks and outcomes to be accomplished during the planning phase and beyond. Although planning is an ongoing effort throughout the project, most of these activities occur here. The schedule, work plan, and contingency and risk plans are just a few documents produced in this phase. The length of these documents, or the decision to combine them into one document, is very dependent on the size of the project.

The execution phase will be described in Chapter 4. The execution phase coordinates the human and nonhuman resources required to carry out the plan. This chapter will outline the processes used to coordinate the activities occurring to complete the project. These processes include managing the work plan tasks and resources, team development, information distribution, and quality assurance. This phase usually occurs concurrently with the controlling phase, which will be described in Chapter 5. The controlling phase ensures that the project objectives are being met and that any variance from the plan can be corrected as necessary. This chapter will outline how the project will be monitored or measured. This is an ongoing process and identifies any variances from what was planned. Processes included during this phase include scope change control, cost control, performance reporting, risk monitoring/control, and schedule control.

The closing phase formalizes the project acceptance and ends it, and it is described in Chapter 6. This chapter will outline the formal process for project acceptance and closure. This phase includes any contract closure required and official review and sign off by the customer. One key step that is often forgotten is to complete all documentation, including lessons learned. These items should be filed away and used as historical information the next time you do a similar project.

Once the phases are described, Chapters 7 and 8 will discuss how to apply the project management process. Chapter 7 will focus on applying the process in healthcare informatics. Clinical informatics is a relatively new field for nurses, and professionals in other clinical specialties, and often includes doing something with data or information technology. The project management process defined in the earlier chapters can be used in the day-to-day life of an Informaticist. This chapter will outline how to apply this methodology to various scenarios or potential projects that a Healthcare Informaticists may face in the workplace.

Chapter 8 will discuss applying the project management process in healthcare management. Healthcare management includes a wide variety of roles from Chief Nursing Officer to Chief Information Officer to department and application level directors. Each of these roles includes projects that must be taken on and successfully managed. This chapter will help to identify these projects and how to apply the methodology described earlier in the book.

Chapter 9 summarizes the project management methodology described earlier in the book, as well as how to apply it to the various roles nurses play in the workforce today. In addition, appendixes will be included. The appendixes will include organizational tips, deliverables templates and examples, project management web sites, and references. These appendixes will help healthcare informaticists find the method that is right for them to stay organized, where they can find additional project management information and sample templates for documents discussed in throughout the book.

The purpose of this book is to serve as a text for healthcare professionals to use when they want to become knowledgeable in project management and/or as a reference if they are currently managing projects.

The anticipated audience for this book includes:

- Staff nurses
- Nurse managers
- Nurse educators
- Staff development instructors
- Advanced practice nurses
- Nurse informaticists
- Researchers
- Analysts
- Department managers
- Consultants
- Physicians
- Therapists
- Pharmacists

Susan M. Houston, MBA, RN-BC, PMP
Lisa Anne Bove, MSN, RN-BC

Acknowledgments

We would like to thank those who have helped us during the writing of this book. Thank you to our families and friends who supported and put up with us while we were working on this book. At times, they encouraged us to continue, whereas at other times, they knew it was best to leave us alone.

Susan would like to send a special thanks to her husband Gary and children Nicole and Matt, who seem to have an unlimited amount of patience.

Lisa sends thanks to her family, for without their support, this would never have happened.

We would both like to thank Patty for providing the extra pair of eyes when a fresh view of the chapters was requested.

It is our pleasure to acknowledge RADM Carol A. Romano, who is a strong supporter of nursing and nursing informatics. We have both had the pleasure of working with RADM Romano and are grateful that she was able to find time in her busy schedule to write our foreword.

Susan M. Houston, MBA, RN-BC, PMP
Lisa Anne Bove, MSN, RN-BC

Contents

Foreword v
    Carol A. Romano

Series Preface vii

Preface ix

Acknowledgments xiii

About the Authors xvii

1. Project Management Process 1

2. Initiation Phase 15

3. Planning Phase 21

4. Execution Phase 35

5. Control Phase 51

6. Closing Phase 63

7. Applying the Project Management Process in
    Healthcare Informatics 69

8. Applying the Project Management Process in
    Healthcare Management 79

9. Summary 91

Bibliography 95

Appendix 99

Index 135

About the Authors

Susan M. Houston, MBA, RN-BC, PMP, and Lisa Anne Bove, MSN, RN-BC, first worked together on an implementation project in a major teaching facility in Maryland. Both authors have extensive project management experience as nurse managers and nurse informaticists. Both authors have used project management principles to successfully manage and complete large, complicated projects. In addition, both authors are currently employed as project managers in health care, one in a hospital setting and one as a software consultant. One author has already achieved PMP certification through the Project Management Institute (PMI) and the other author has internal company project manager certification and is completing the necessary prework to sit for the PMI project manger exam. Both authors are also certified by the American Nurses Credentialing Center in Nursing Informatics and hold master's degrees.

Susan M. Houston started working in an emergency room while in nursing school. After graduation, she continued to work in emergency medicine for over 15 years, finishing as a nurse manager of a level 2 trauma center. Susan was asked to implement a clinical information system because she was one of the few nurses who were comfortable with computers. This began her career as a project manager, implementing clinical systems. Susan has worked for a software vendor, implementing a wide range of applications for their clients. Susan has also worked as a consultant, implementing new processes and systems for a variety of healthcare organizations. Susan has a master's degree in business administration.

Susan is currently the Vice President for the Project Management Institute's Healthcare Specific Interest Group (SIG). She was a charter member of this SIG, and has been on the board of directors for this organization since 2005. Susan is also on the faculty at the University of Maryland Baltimore School of Nursing, where she teaches an Information Technology Project Management course for the Master's of Nursing Informatics program. Susan has also presented at several conferences, as well as coauthored several articles. In her current role, Susan has developed and is managing the Project Management Office at a large teaching research hospital, implementing several large and small projects while mentoring other project managers.

Lisa Anne Bove started as a critical care nurse in a major teaching facility in Philadelphia. After completing her master's as a critical care clinical specialist, Lisa Anne worked as a staff development instructor and clinical nurse specialist. As such, she managed projects that included developing critical care courses,

GN to RN programs, and Joint Commission on Accreditation of Healthcare Organizations mandated training programs, orientation programs, and research projects. She got involved in healthcare informatics when the hospital she was working for implemented order entry and results reporting throughout the hospital. She served on the user committees, and then moved into the informatics department to start as an analyst and database administrator. As an analyst, Lisa Anne implemented many applications, including an OR system and an inventory management system, and assisted with other system upgrades and extensions.

Lisa Anne then began to work for a software vendor, first as a trainer and then as a project manger. In these roles, Lisa Anne managed many projects, including developing new training programs, large facility implementation projects, and clinical beta implementation projects.

In her current position as a consultant, Lisa Anne manages a variety of implementation and process redesign projects across the country. She is currently on the Board of Directors of the American Nursing Informatics Association (ANIA) and a member of the Healthcare Information Management Systems Society (HIMSS) Nursing Informatics Taskforce. Lisa Anne has published on both nursing and informatics topics and speaks frequently at nursing conferences both locally and internationally.

1
Project Management Process

Introduction

The project management process defines how a project should be managed to decrease the risk of failure. Using a consistent methodology to manage all projects is one of the most important steps toward project success. The methodology provides a standard way of managing projects that is used consistently across all projects and ensures that all aspects of the project are considered, evaluated, and documented. This helps to improve the success of all projects. There are defined phases each project goes through: initiation, planning, execution and control, and, finally, closure. Each phase has defined activities for the project manager, the project team, and the project stakeholders. The duration of the phases may also vary between projects, as well as within projects, but each project spends some time in each phase.

The project management process is a defined methodology that can be used to manage projects large or small. Although the phases of the process are generally consistent across industries, the specific method of moving through the phases may differ from one organization to another. This process may even have different names, including project management life cycle, project management methodology, or project management framework. The Project Management Institute (www.pmi.org) identifies five process groups or phases. The five phases are initiating, planning, executing, controlling, and closing. An overview of these phases will be presented in this chapter, followed by a closer examination of each in the subsequent chapters. Before the phases are reviewed, it is important to understand the difference between a project and a process, as well as the concept of the triple constraint (Figure 1.1).

Project Versus Process

What is a project and how does it differ from a process? A project has a defined beginning and end, such as the implementation of an application or the development of a training program. A process is an ongoing activity, such as

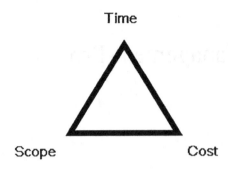

FIGURE 1.1. Triple constraint.

support and maintenance of an application or the offering of an ongoing training program. A project is temporary. A process is continuous. A project needs to be managed to ensure it is completed on time and within budget, while meeting the defined need. A process needs to be managed to ensure compliance and to continuously improve as needed. Resources are assigned to a project for a defined time frame to complete specific activities. Resources work on processes as part of their ongoing work effort. Each project is unique, although some are similar enough that they can provide historical information to assist with initiation and planning of other projects (Tables 1.1 and 1.2).

TABLE 1.1. Project versus process.

Project	Process
Defined beginning and end	Ongoing activity
Temporary	Continuous
Managed to time, budget, and need	Managed to compliance and continuous improvement
Resources assigned for specific time frame	Resources are ongoing

TABLE 1.2. What is a project?

It is temporary	Has a defined start and finish
It is unique	Develops a new product or service
It is progressive	Proceeds in steps or on a specific plan
It is elaborated	Worked out with care, coordination, and detail

The Triple Constraint

Every project is constrained in some way by scope, cost, and time. These limitations are known as the triple constraint. These are often competing goals, and they need to be balanced by the project manager throughout the project life cycle. Scope is related to the work that needs to be done and what is expected by the customer at the end of the project. Cost is related to the budget or how much money will be required to complete the project. Time is related to the duration of project or the schedule.

The project manager should consider the triple constraint while planning for the project and analyze any modifications requested or required during all phases of the project. Any modification to the project will impact one or more of these three constraints, and will often require trade offs between them. If there is an increase in scope, either cost or time will be impacted. Either additional resources (cost) will be required to meet the deadline (time) or the schedule (time) will need to be extended if the team resources (cost) remain the same. A project manager needs to understand which aspect of the triple constraint is the most important and cannot be impacted, as well as which one can be modified as needed. The priorities of the triple constraint are usually defined by the sponsors during the initiation and planning phases.

The Project Management Process

Initiation Phase

The initiation phase is the first phase of the project management process. It is during this phase that the project is selected and defined. The business's need, goals, and objectives define what the project needs to accomplish and why it is being done. Once the business's need, goals, and objectives are determined, historical information from similar past projects should be reviewed. The historical information is beneficial in further definition and planning. The project manager should review information about resources, budget, and task information, as well as lessons learned from all similar projects. This provides the project manager with a place to start to plan this project.

Identification of stakeholders is another important task for the project manager during the initiation phase. Stakeholder involvement early in the process helps to obtain their buy-in throughout the project. Stakeholders are any people with an interest in the project. This includes the business owners, project team members, project sponsors, end-users, and any other internal customers that will be affected by the project or the project deliverables. If there are a large number of end-users, a few representatives should be selected to act as stakeholders. The stakeholders are involved in defining the high-level deliverables, constraints, assumptions, and measures of success, as well as time, cost, and resource estimates for the project.

The strategy for managing the project should also be discussed with the stakeholders during the initiation phase. If the organization has a standard project management methodology, it should be reviewed to ensure all understand and will agree to follow the process. The responsibilities of the project manager should also be reviewed and/or defined. It is important for all stakeholders and team members to understand the project manager's authority and accountability.

Once all of this information is collected and verified with the stakeholders, it is documented in a project charter or project scope. These documents provide details about the definition of the project, including scope, constraints, project team members, and project manager authority. The project sponsors are the senior level stakeholders who are identified to make decisions regarding the scope and are available for issue resolution when they need to be escalated beyond the project manager. The sponsor, or sponsors, should include someone from the business impacted by the project and/or someone from the IT department if it is an IT project. For example, if you were implementing a new admission/discharge/transfer (ADT) system, the sponsors would be the Director of Admissions and the Chief Information Officer. The sponsors are asked to sign off on these documents to provide formal approval to move forward to the next phase, which is planning.

Planning Phase

The planning phase is the most important phase of the project management process, and it should not be rushed. This phase is where decisions are made about how to complete the project and accomplish the goals and objectives defined in the initiation phase. If there is a standard project management methodology in place at the organization, this phase is made easier. Plans, such as a scope management plan, can and should be reused for all projects. If these are in place already, they do not need to be created from scratch. The utilization of historical information from previous projects allows the project manager to have a head start on some planning. Reviewing the communication plan or the identified risks from previous plans provides some valuable information moving into a new project.

The planning phase ends with a kickoff meeting for all project stakeholders. This is where the project plans are all reviewed and validated. Ensuring all project team members have the same information before beginning their activities helps to increase the project's chances for success. The approval of the project plan closes this phase and, as some say, the "real work" of the project begins with the next phases.

Execution and Control Phases

The execution and control phases occur concurrently, but the activities are different. During the execution phase, the project progress is managed and all project plans are executed. In other words, what the team said they would do in planning is done in execution. In the controlling phase, the project performance is measured and controlled. The project performance includes scope change, quality control, and risk control.

These two phases are usually the longest in the project process. The project manager needs to make sure the project happens as planned and to take corrective action when any variances occur. Information distribution is often the largest part of the project manager's role, as they are the hub for all communication coming into the team and going out to the stakeholders. The project plans should be updated regularly and modified as needed, until the project reaches the closing phase.

Closing

The closing phase is the last phase of the project. This is where the final verification occurs to ensure that what was produced by the project is what the team set out to produce. Final analysis of scope, cost, and time is completed and documented. The sponsors accept the project deliverables and agree and sign-off that the project is completed to their satisfaction. Lessons learned are documented as an important step to assist with future projects. Once all records are finalized and archived, the resources can be released to move onto other projects or other work, and the project is officially completed (Table 1.3).

TABLE 1.3. Project management process.

Initiation	Planning	Execution	Controlling	Closing
Select a Project	Determine project team	Execute the project plan	Scope change control	Procurement audit
Determine goals and objectives	Develop work plan	Manage project progress	Risk monitoring and control	Project verification
Review historical information	Estimate time and cost	Distribute information	Corrective action	Lessons learned
Determine high-level deliverables, constraints, assumptions	Identify risks, mitigation strategies, and risk management plan	Quality assurance	Project performance measuring	End of project performance reporting
Define project manager's authority	Develop budget and budget plan	Hold status meetings	Quality control	Update and archive all records
Finalize project charter/scope document	Define all other Plans (training, communication implementation, etc.)	Identify changes	Ensure compliance with plans	Formal acceptance
	Finalize project plan and Obtain approval		Cost and schedule control	Celebrate
	Kickoff meeting			Release resources

Project Management Office (PMO)

Many organizations have created a project management office to provide best practices and support for managing projects. A PMO is an organizational group responsible for the coordination of all projects managed in an organization. A PMO should provide a standard methodology for managing projects, including standardized plans and document templates. The office can also provide education, coaching, and mentoring, as well as project management resources. Although PMOs have been around for quite some time in other industries, they are relatively new to healthcare. With the federal directive for increased healthcare information technology, the industry has begun the challenging task of implementing more and more information technology systems. With this increase in projects, there is a greater need for project management and consistent methodology for managing projects.

Several roles may be included in a PMO. The Director/Manager of the PMO provides the leadership and direction for the office. Other roles include project managers, project team leaders, business analysts, and support staff. While these roles are important for managing projects, some staff may perform multiple roles by choice or because there are not enough staff to separate them. Some PMOs may choose not to include some roles, such as project team leader or systems analyst, because they are not required. Table 1.4 lists the role, responsibilities, and expected skills and background for these suggested PMO roles.

TABLE 1.4. The Roles in a PMO.

Role	Responsibility	Skills and Background
Director PMO	• Reports to Senior C-level Executive. • Provides leadership, direction, and support for projects under development and execution, ensuring that all projects have clear goals, objectives, timelines, and measurable milestones. • Oversees development and management of the Project Office. • Promotes the development and diffusion of project management culture. • Maintains effective communication with senior management. • Oversees education, coaching, and mentoring for staff related to project management. • Maintains an understanding of current project management techniques and industry practices. • Identifies project interrelationships that will affect priority and resource allocation decisions. • Monitors project milestones, schedules, resource constraints, etc., and updates senior management as necessary. • With functional and project managers, analyzes the impact to existing projects of additional projects or changes to current projects and identifies strategies for accomplishing all desired projects • Responsible for the overall project management function • Provides coordination, support and management to PMO processes and activities • Creates and maintains a uniform approach to project management and serves as change agent for continuous improvement through improved/enhanced methodologies.	• Ability to analyze and synthesize information in a concise manner. • Ability to understand and deal with political issues in a matrix environment. • Excellent communication skills and creditability with executive management. • Strong organizational skills and the ability to manage multiple priorities. • Strong leadership ability and negotiation skills. • Strong skills in conflict resolution and problem solving. • Willingness to assume responsibility for making recommendations for critical decisions related to projects. • Ability to instill trust in, motivate, and work with others. • Customer and results oriented. • Thorough understanding of budgeting and resource mgmt. • Extensive knowledge of project management tools and methodologies, as well as project management and business management software. • Experience with rollout of project management and process improvement in an organization. • Ability to manage large, complex projects on time and within budget. • Ability to express complex technical concepts effectively to a diverse group of people. • 7–10 years project management experience.

(Continued)

TABLE 1.4. **(Continued)**

Role	Responsibility	Skills and Background
	• Oversees the project management strategy, training, communication, project control/analysis/reporting, process, and tool development. • Provides recommendations for the appointment of project managers. • Assists with approval of scope, schedule, resources, roles, and issue resolution for projects as necessary. • Oversees risk management process. • Maintains the master status list of all projects and provides "dashboard" reports and analysis to senior leadership. • Facilitates resolution of multi-project resource and integration conflicts.	• PMP or other project management certification or equivalent experience. • MBA or equivalent.
Project Manager	• Manages cross-functional teams responsible for delivering defined project outputs on time, within budget, and with quality results • Plan, organize, monitor, and oversee one or more projects to meet defined requirements or specifications. • Primary responsibility to defining, planning, tracking, and managing the project, for identifying key resources and providing the direction they require to meet the project objectives. • Ensure the appropriate management, customer, and supplier involvement throughout the life of the project. • May not have direct supervisory responsibility for team members, but provides performance input to their functional managers. • May be responsible for one or more projects. • Negotiate the performance of activities with team members and their managers in a matrix environment. • Coach to clarify assignments and deliverables, mentor others in project management practices, and review quality of work.	• Knowledge and competency in project management processes, including planning tasks and allocating resources; risk, issue, time, and quality management; monitoring and reporting; working in teams; documentation; and record keeping. • Ability to plan and facilitate meetings. • Strategic, conceptual analytical thinking, and decision-making skills. • Adaptability and flexibility, including ability to manage deadline pressure, ambiguity, and change. • Negotiating skills. • Presentation and written communication skills. • Ability to advise on complex matters to nonspecialists. • Personal integrity and courage to escalate issues about project to management when necessary and to advocate for responsible solutions to project problems.

- Manage and communicate a clear vision of the project objectives and motivate the team to achieve them.
- Organize the work into manageable activity clusters (phases) and determine an effective approach to completing the work.
- Prepare project plan and obtain management approval.
- Manage relationships with stakeholders and project team.
- Manage change to preserve plan commitments and initiate review if objectives must change.
- Establish and communicate clear priorities among project activities.
- Arbitrate and resolve conflict and problems within the project.
- Ensure all project documentation is completed throughout the life of the project
- Effectively coordinate the activities of the team to meet project milestones
- Represents project in meetings to ensure priorities are communicated and understood and that progress/delays/issues are reported
- Determines what constitutes successful closure for all parties and gain acceptance and sign-off when closure is attained

- Extensive knowledge of project management methodology.
- Exceptional interpersonal skills, the ability to work well with people from different disciplines with clear, concise, and tactful communication.
- Analyze risks, establish contingency plans, and identify trigger events and responsibility for initiating mitigation activities.
- Responsible for project problem/issue identification and resolution.
- Track and report on progress to plan, cost, and schedule as well as change control.
- Analyze the actual performance against the plan and make adjustments consistent with the plan objectives.
- Ability to build teams and generate a spirit of cooperation, while coordinating diverse activities.
- Demonstrated expertise in creating and maintaining project deliverables, issues, scope, and quality, while bringing projects to successful completion within the cost and time requirements.
- 3–5 years using formal project management methodologies, techniques, and tools.
- PMP and/or other industry and project management certification.
- College degree, preferably in industry or equivalent work experience.

(Continued)

TABLE 1.4. (Continued)

Role	Responsibility	Skills and Background
Project Team Leader	• Is a senior staff member appointed by the project manager to lead a sub-project group, to supervise and represent a team within a larger project • May be responsible for one or more sub-project components • Define, plan, track and managing the sub-project, and providing the direction the team requires to meet the project objectives • Manage and communicate a clear vision of the project objectives and motivate the team to achieve them • Prepare sub-project plan and obtain PM approval • Track and report on progress to plan • Ensure all sub-project documentation is completed throughout the life of the project • Effectively coordinate the activities of the team to meet project milestones • Regularly reports status to project manager • Escalates issues to project manager for resolution if necessary	• Should posses a subset of the skills and experience necessary to be a project manager • Knowledge of the principles and practices of project management. • Conceptual and analytical thinking skills. • Decision making and problem-solving skills. • Adaptability and flexibility including ability to manage pressure, ambiguity, and change. • General management skills necessary to plan, organize, and prioritize workload. • Communication skills required for reporting on progress and leading meetings.
Project Budget Coordinator	• Track project performance against budgets, plans and schedules • Managing the integration of multiple programs and projects • Providing data, analysis and reporting to the project managers and various levels of management • Provide input and review for the development of schedule, WBS, estimates and work packages during different phases of the project • Maintain accurate records of committed, expended and forecast costs and monitor project costs and EVM measurements • Review time and cost impacts for any requested changes to scope • Manage the cost, financial and procurement data • Apply appropriate metrics and tools for project control • Identify cost-savings opportunities and develop programs to achieve long term savings	• Sound task management skills and strong analytical ability. • Strong communication skills. • Strong attention to detail and organizational skills. • Ability to work effectively as a member of a team and foster teamwork in others. • Demonstrated ability to handle multiple concurrent assignments. • Advanced computer skills and knowledge of the current industry standard applications. • Ability to perform comprehensive organizational forecasting and analysis. • Ability to work in a flexible team environment and independently with minimal supervision.

- High-level analytical skills and management accounting knowledge.
- Experience summarizing results and producing project management reports.
- Experience in budgeting, forecasting, scheduling, and analytical reporting, including baseline development and EVM systems.
- 5–10 yrs experience in PM role, greater than 5 yrs in planning/scheduling/controlling functions.
- PMP or other project management certification.
- Certification in costs and/or contract management a plus.
- Strong communication skills.
- Full proficiency with relevant software tools.
- Ability to work in cross-functional team environment.
- Must be a team player and demonstrate a teamwork approach to performance.
- Good time management and organizational skills.
- Sound understanding of project management processes.
- Experience developing project plans, including WBS, project schedules, and resource planning and leveling.

Project Planner/Scheduler

- Assists project managers and by developing, analyzing and managing project plans, schedules and resource forecasts
- Prepare and keep current master project plans as well as sub-project plans
- Develop WBS, critical path, schedules, resources and project timelines
- Perform critical path analysis and develop timelines for completing of tasks
- Update master and sub-project plans with new information as changes occur and monitor dependencies affected by these changes
- Responsible for communicating any schedule conflicts, resource constraints and time constraints to the project manager and Director/Manager of PMO
- Communicate and publish plans to appropriate involved individuals
- Provide planning and resource allocation services that support the project schedule
- Support the preparation of progress reports, standardized reporting procedures an the monitoring of overall project performance

(Continued)

TABLE 1.4. (Continued)

Role	Responsibility	Skills and Background
Project Office Administrator/ Knowledge Mgmt Coordinator	• Assist project managers with administrative duties • Maintain procedures, tools and practices of PMO • Control revisions to scope, schedule and other project documents • Obtain required signatures for project documentation • Assist with project management training coordination and meeting planning and management • Maintain and monitor issue logs across projects • Scribing notes at project meetings • Support communication plans • Maintains the repository for all project historical documents • Update project management websites, intranet or community practice tool • Assist with developing written processes, procedures and flowcharts to support PMO activities • Facilitate communication within the team by ensuring accessibility and completeness of information	• Excellent communication skills. • Attention to detail. • Effectively working independently, as well as part of a team. • Ability to multitask. • Detail oriented and flexible. • Good prioritization, time management, and organizational skills. • Understanding of project management principles and practices. • 3–5 years experience in industry. • Project management training required. • Expert skill level with relevant software applications.
Contract Officer	• All contract negotiation and coordination • Resolution of all contract issues • Maintains all contract documentation • Contract change management	• NIH Project Officer training (Basic and Advanced). • Federal Government Contract Warrants.
Business Analyst	• Define and document business needs and requirements • Generate business cases	• Strong business background with knowledge of industry. • Skilled writer and communicator. • Good communication and presentation skills. • Knowledge of project management principles and practices. • Business and project management education and training. • 3–5 years experience in industry.

Systems Analyst	• Analyzes, designs and develops information systems to support project manager and acts as subject matter expert in project management technology	• Ability to understand project management technology and best practices. as well as the ability to learn and apply new technology/tools quickly.
	• Customize, configure and troubleshoot software to support project management methodology and practice	• Good communication skills.
	• Develop and deploy enterprise project control tools, procedures and systems	• Proficiency in a wider range of project management and productivity tools.
	• Define and document technical requirements	• Ability to work in teams.
		• Teaching or coaching ability a plus, but not required.

2
Initiation Phase

Introduction

The initiation phase is the first step in the project management process. This phase is where the project begins to be defined, is authorized, and links the project work to the organizational strategic objectives. The deliverable for this phase is the project charter, which defines the project and provides authorization to do the project once approved by the project sponsors. Many of the things that are initially defined in this phase are further refined later in the process. The identified assumptions and constraints will feed into the planning that will occur in the next phase. These tend to lead into risks and contingency planning. High-level deliverables and resource needs are further defined as the work plan is developed.

Project Selection

Project management begins with selecting a project. Many organizations have a list of strategic initiatives they would like to accomplish. These may include improved access to patient medical records, decreasing patient length of stay, or improved billing accuracy. Some of these initiatives will include completing a project. Even the implementation of a new or revised process can be a project if there is a clear delineation of when the project is completed, allowing the new process to continue. A level of analysis occurs before the selection of which initiatives will be accomplished at this time and which projects will be supported. The initiation phase may be completed on several projects to clearly understand the scope and estimated cost of each. Once the project charter has been created and evaluated, it may be accepted, and the project continues, or it may be denied or deferred to another time. Resources are limited, whether human or financial, and some organizations are unable to accomplish all the projects they want in a given time frame. The information gathered during this phase and outlined in the project charter helps senior leadership make an educated decision on which projects should continue. A project manager should be identified as early in the process as possible to allow for consistency in leadership. If this is not possible, someone should be identified to create the project charter and hand off to the project manager.

Historical Information

Historical information is information that currently exists related to past projects. This information may include any project documentation, including charters, lessons learned, issue lists, work plans, etc. Evaluating the documentation from previous projects that are similar to the new one, or that utilize similar resources, can help give the project manager a better understanding of what may occur during the current project. Issue lists from a previous project could help in evaluating potential risks and mitigation strategies. The work plans can provide information about the initial expected tasks to be completed and what was actually necessary to complete the project. These documents alone can provide valuable information regarding what tasks are required, how long they actually took to complete and who can do them. Previous plans, such as the risk management plan and the communication plan, can also provide information to be considered as the project manager defines the project. Other sources of historical information include meeting minutes from the board of directors, steering committees, or department meetings, as well as documented organizational goals, objectives, and plans for the future.

The information from these sources can be used by the project manager during the initiating and planning phases of the project lifecycle. The information that may be helpful includes the following:

- Identified risks and their mitigation strategies.
- Lessons learned document, including what went right, what went wrong, and what could be done better in the future.
- Time and cost estimates, as well as the final project duration and cost.
- Communication plan.
- Initial and final project plans, tasks, durations, and resources.

Business Need, Project Goal, and Objectives

An analysis of the business need helps to define the reason for doing the project. The needs analysis is where the project begins to be defined. During the needs analysis tasks, the project should be defined by answering the following questions:

- Why do we want to do this project?
- What will happen if the project is not done?
- What are the benefits of doing the project?
- What are the risks of not doing the project?

The project goal is the outcome of the project, or final state desired after the project is complete. The project objectives help to define specifics within the goal. While the goal and objectives are being defined, they need to be matched up to the organizational goals and objectives to avoid conflicts. The objectives should also be evaluated for conflicts between themselves. Conflicting objectives occur when input is provided by multiple departments or areas within the organization that have differing views of the purpose of the project. These conflicts need to be resolved before moving on, and your sponsors can assist.

A business need could be "The ability to have access to the patient medical record wherever and whenever it is needed." This could lead to a goal of "To provide access to the patient medical record to all authorized staff from any workstation on campus." This goal could lend itself to the following objectives:

- The medical records will be available electronically on any workstation on campus.
- The medical records will be secured to allow access only by those authorized.
- The available medical records will include the most current information and will be updated continuously.

Current State Documentation

An important step during the initiation phase is to document the current state. This is what is currently in place related to the goals and objectives of the project. In the example above, the current state would include how the medical record is accessed by authorized staff and how is it viewed, updated, and stored for future access. Documenting the current state usually is summarized as a flow diagram. Some examples include how orders are documented and processed or how medications are documented. Although project managers and teams often skip this step, current state documentation is very important to assist the project team with future state planning. Future state should also be documented. This is what will be in place in relation to the goals and objectives after the project is complete. This is usually done through the goals and objectives of the project. By defining the current state and the future state, it becomes clear what the project needs to accomplish. If the future state includes any changes in processes these should also be documented. This step can also be called process redesign. Any project causes changes to current state and creates a future state. Some changes are small, but some changes can be huge or change multiple processes for multiple users. Using the example above, the way the end user documents their orders or medications given will change. Project managers need to understand what the new processes will look like and how the users will be affected by the change. For best results, the staff in the area impacted need to be involved in the process redesign effort or they will not buy into the results. Meetings should be held with a group of end users to help define the current state. Once the project is approved, these same users can assist with documenting the new processes.

These user groups can be an asset as the project progresses. They represent the end users and can help the project team through planning, process redesign, user acceptance testing, and training.

Project Charter

The project charter is the document that defines, and when approved, authorizes the project. Needs assessment, goals, objectives, current state, and future state are all included in this document. Additional information that should be in the charter includes high-level deliverables, high-level estimates of resources and costs, potential constraints, and assumptions. The project charter is the baseline document for later phases of the project to assess progress, further define process, and to evaluate changes to the project.

With the goal and objectives defined, the project manager facilitates the definition of what is in scope and out of scope, i.e., what will be done and what will not. With the previous example, the scope could be defined as:

- Implement an electronic medical record.
- Include an interface to the Lab system.
- Do not include an interface to the radiology system until a future phase.

The high-level deliverables define what will actually be delivered at the end of the project. What is the output or tangible item that will be delivered when the project is over? This could include a new software package, a new process being followed, or new hardware deployed on patient care units. High-level estimates also need to be defined. Historical documentation helps a great deal with this portion of the charter. Because charters are written early in the project, there are still a lot of unknowns, and estimations of resources and costs are difficult. Reviewing previous projects that are similar can help with the estimates, even if they are only slightly similar. If another project includes interfaces, for example, the documentation can assist with the estimation of the interface portion of this project related to the necessary resources, time commitment, and cost for doing an interface. The estimates for human resources should include all aspects of the project. For a software implementation project, these estimates could include business analysts, systems analysts, system developers, database administrators, network administrators, testers, trainers, and help desk support staff. The project manager should look at the human resources available within the organization and evaluate whether contract staff are required to fill in gaps in expertise. If needed, contract staff should be included in the estimations. Will a single project manager be used to manage the project? If the project is large, project team leaders may be used to manage sections of the project. An example could be a technical project team leader who manages all technical aspects of the project, including hardware procurement and configuration, networking, and interfaces. Each project team leader would then report to the project manager on all tasks related to their area of responsibility.

TABLE 2.1. Risk assessment and mitigation strategy.

Risk	Mitigation Strategy
There may be a delay in procuring the hardware, which may impact the time scheduled for hardware configuration.	1. Monitor the procurement process closely with frequent updates from hardware vendor. 2. Review hardware configuration activity to see if the schedule can be shortened if necessary.

Any known assumptions or constraints should also be included in the project charter. Assumptions are the things that are assumed to be true to plan the project. Assumptions could include items such as "the funds will be available to complete the project as defined," "contractors will be used for testing and training activities," or "all end users will be trained to use the system within six weeks of go-live." Constraints are the things that restrict what can be done on the project. Constraints may include items such as "the project must be completed in nine months," "the budget is limited to phase 1, and phase 2 will require a new funding source before beginning," or "the new application must be able to run on the current workstations." Both assumptions and constraints are important to define, and may lead to known risks.

Risks are things that can jeopardize the project's success. Identifying known risks happens at the beginning of a project and is reassessed throughout the project. Risks can be identified by reviewing the historical documentation, constraints, assumptions, and estimations discussed earlier. Once a risk is identified, a mitigation strategy should be noted to try and avoid or limit the effect of the risk (Table 2.1).

The project timeline may be dependent on the constraints or interproject dependencies. There may be requirements that the project is completed in a specific time frame or it cannot begin until after another project is complete. These dependencies, along with available resources, funding, and historical information will all play a role in defining the project's timeline, when it will begin, and the estimated completion date.

Project Scope Document

The project scope document is a less formal document that defines the project and authorizes it, when approved. Depending on the formality of the organization and the size of the project, a scope document could be completed in place of a more formal charter. Much of the same information can be included in the scope document, but it tends to be shorter and more concise. If the project is small, additional information such as communication and risk strategies can be included in the scope document rather than in separate plans. Small projects tend to be shorter in duration or smaller in scope where there is much less documentation is required. The project scope document still authorizes the project and should be signed by the sponsors.

Roles and Responsibilities

The responsibilities and authority of the project manager should be defined during the initiation phase. This allows the project manager to move into the planning phase with a good understanding of the boundaries of their role on the project. The project manager will need to get some guidance on who the stakeholders and sponsors are. Stakeholders are the people who have some interest in or are affected by the project. Sponsors are the people who are champions for the project, they have the authority to resolve issues that need to be escalated, approve the scope of the project, requirements, and any requested changes. The sponsors also accept the final deliverables and accept the project as being complete. There may be one or more sponsors on a project, but they should be kept to a minimum. For example, the implementation of a new pharmacy system, the sponsors might be the CIO and the head of the pharmacy department.

Summary

During the initiation phase, the project manager creates the document that defines and authorizes the project. Project charter and scope documents support the project's goals and objectives and assist the project team and stakeholders to maintain focus.

3
Planning Phase

Introduction

Planning is defining and refining objectives and selecting the best course of action to accomplish the project objectives. During the initiation phase, quite a bit of information was gathered to help define the project. The project charter or scope documents, which provided validation and approval for the project, were completed. During the planning phase, the approach to accomplish the project is defined. This includes defining the necessary tasks or activities, the resources, the schedule, and the budget. Research demonstrates that good planning is associated with project success, even though senior management and team members are often impatient to begin work on the project and see results. The deliverable of this phase is a comprehensive project plan that is approved by the sponsors and shared with the entire team in a project kickoff meeting.

Planning

Some management gurus feel good planning never cuts the implementation time and is not necessary for good business. Planning is the most important step in the project lifecycle. The majority of project management gurus feel that if problems arise during the life of a project, the cause can usually be tracked back to the lack of planning. Without planning, team members will not know what is expected of them or when it is expected, team members will not know what to do when an expected risk arises and may waste valuable time dealing with what to do. Because planning is the most important step does not mean that all project management is planning; the amount of planning is equivalent to the scope of the project. It is difficult to determine exactly how much time should be spent on planning because of the many variables involved. The more information available to assist with planning, the shorter the planning phase will be. If there is a standard project management methodology in place, with standard plans used across projects, less time will be needed to document these plans than if they needed to be created from scratch. The quantity of historical information available from similar projects will also assist to shorten the length of time on planning.

The project plan that is defined in this phase is actually made up of many plans. Some of these are defined specifically for this project, such as the work plan, whereas others should be standard plans utilized consistently across all projects, such as the scope management plan. Understanding the interdependencies between plans is necessary to ensure all are coordinated, consistent, and accurate. If there is a change to one plan, another plan may need to be modified based on new information. All of these plans go through multiple iterations until they are final and approved by the sponsors. They are also reevaluated throughout the project.

Project Team

The high-level project resources have already been defined in the initiation phase. The project manager needs to work with the organization to identify the actual team members based on these projected resource needs. Who in the organization the project manager works with to have staff assigned will depend on the organizational structure. In functional and matrix organizations, the project manager will need to work with the staff's manager to identify who is available and when they are available to work on this project. In project organizations, the project staff report to the project manager, and a balance between projects is necessary rather than negotiation with managers to identify team members.

Functional organizations are the most common. This organization is grouped by areas of specialty or function, such as finance, marketing, and manufacturing. In healthcare organizations, these may include finance, information technology, inpatient care, and outpatient care. Communication occurs up and down in the silos, and usually not horizontally (Figure 3.1).

Matrix organizations attempt to maximize the strengths and minimize the weaknesses of the functional and project formats. Team members report to two bosses, their functional manager and the project manager for the project they are currently working on. In a strong matrix organization, the power rests with the project manager. In a weak matrix organization the power is with the functional

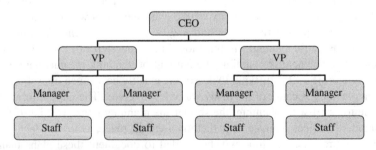

FIGURE 3.1. Functional organization.

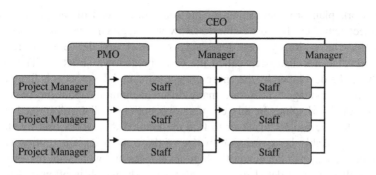

FIGURE 3.2. Matrix organization.

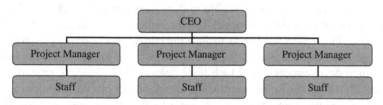

FIGURE 3.3. Project organization.

manager. A balanced matrix organization has power shared equally between the two managers. A healthcare organization with a project management office (PMO) may function in this manor (Figure 3.2).

Project organizations have staff aligned with their projects. The project manager has total control of the projects and their resources. This type of organization, e.g., a consulting company, typically only does projects (Figure 3.3).

Once the team is identified, it is important to remember that the actual resource requirements may change as the project activities are further defined. The project manager should be able to work closely with the team member's managers as the work is planned, task durations and timing are defined, and if the resources need to be modified. This working relationship continues throughout the project, as the work is continuously evaluated in relation to risks, issues, and approved changes. The project manager is the leader of the team and needs to inspire and motivate the team to achieve the project goals.

Work Plan

The work plan is often called the project plan. It is the listing of all activities with durations, start and finish dates, and resources, and it is often created using specific software, such as Microsoft Project. The work plan is only part of the entire project plan.

The work plan provides a map of the route to the end of the project, and the project manager should be able to know at any given time what work and deliverables have already been done and what work and deliverables are left. The work plan has also been called the work breakdown structure. The work plan should be developed by the entire project team, and the process is facilitated by the project manager. There are many different opinions about the best way to create the work plan. In this chapter, two options will be discussed. It is important for the project manager to find the method that works best for them, and it will probably be a variation of one of these methods. One option is for the project manager to document the high-level tasks and work with the specific team members to add detail to each high-level task, which is often called the top-down method. Another option is to get the entire team together to define the tasks in a brainstorming activity.

The project manager should be able to document the high-level tasks for the project based on previous experience and the information collected in the initiation phase. These high-level tasks include the initial tasks of development of the charter or scope document and its approval, initial team identification, and initial project plan development. Other high-level tasks could include the procurement and installation of hardware or software, development or configuration of the application, testing, training, and activation activities. Once these are identified, the team members who will be involved with each area provide the details of the activities to be included (Figure 3.4).

	☉	Task Name	Work	Duration	Start	Finish	% Complete	Predecessors	Resource Names
1		⊟ Device Deployment	1,589.92 hrs	174 days	Tue 4/1/03	Fri 11/28/03	33%		
2	✓	Creation of Initial Deployment Team	7.92 hrs	11 days	Tue 4/1/03	Tue 4/15/03	100%		Sue[9%]
3	✓	⊞ Deployment Plan	322 hrs	22 days	Wed 4/16/03	Thu 5/15/03	100%		
9		⊟ New Device Planning	144 hrs	52 days	Wed 4/23/03	Thu 7/3/03	74%		
10	✓	Meet w/Depts For Device Quantities	60 hrs	20 days	Wed 4/23/03	Tue 5/20/03	100%	2FS+5 days	Sue[38%]
11	✓	Present Budget for Approval	1 hr	1 day	Wed 5/21/03	Wed 5/21/03	100%	10	Jane[13%]
12	✓	Approval of Budget	4 hrs	1 day	Thu 5/22/03	Thu 5/22/03	100%	11	Larry[50%]
13	✓	Finalize Device Quantities	8 hrs	4 days	Fri 5/23/03	Wed 5/28/03	100%	12	Jane[13%],Sue[13%]
14	✓	Finalize Pricing with Vendors	8 hrs	10 days	Thu 5/29/03	Wed 6/11/03	100%	13	Jane[10%]
15	✓	Finalize Delivery Schedule	12 hrs	10 days	Thu 6/12/03	Wed 6/25/03	100%	14	Barry[15%]
16	✓	Approval for Purchase	4 hrs	1 day	Thu 6/26/03	Thu 6/26/03	100%	14,15	Steve[50%]
17	✓	Device Purchase	16 hrs	5 days	Fri 6/27/03	Thu 7/3/03	100%	16	Jeff[40%]
18		Finalize Device Image	20 hrs	10 days	Mon 5/12/03	Wed 6/6/03	0%	6	Barry[25%]
19		Receive & Prep Demo Device	1 hr	2 days	Mon 6/23/03	Wed 6/25/03	0%	18FS+3 days	Jim[6%]
20		Configure Demo Device with Image	8 hrs	5 days	Wed 6/25/03	Wed 7/2/03	0%	19	Chris[20%]
21		Demo Image for Approval	2 hrs	1 day	Thu 7/3/03	Thu 7/3/03	0%	20	Steve[25%]
22		⊞ Printing	260 hrs	165 days	Tue 4/8/03	Fri 11/28/03	16%		
30		⊟ Deployment of New Devices	768 hrs	118 days	Tue 4/8/03	Thu 9/18/03	0%		
31		⊟ Shipment 1	137 hrs	10 days	Fri 8/15/03	Thu 8/28/03	0%	17FS+30 days	
32		Receive & Verify Image	50 hrs	5 days	Fri 8/15/03	Thu 8/21/03	0%		Jim[63%],Leo[63%]
33		Deliver & Configure	75 hrs	5 days	Fri 8/15/03	Thu 8/21/03	0%		Jim[47%],Harry[47%]
34		Surplus Old Devices	12 hrs	5 days	Fri 8/22/03	Thu 8/28/03	0%	33	Jane[30%]
35		⊞ Shipment 2	175 hrs	10 days	Fri 8/22/03	Thu 9/4/03	0%		
39		⊞ Shipment 3	175 hrs	10 days	Fri 8/29/03	Thu 9/11/03	0%		
43		⊞ Shipment 4	175 hrs	10 days	Fri 9/5/03	Thu 9/18/03	0%		
47		Redeployment of Testing Devices	22 hrs	10 days	Tue 4/8/03	Mon 4/21/03	0%		Jim[14%],Joe[14%]
48		Redeployment of Training Devices	84 hrs	15 days	Tue 4/8/03	Mon 4/28/03	0%		Jim[35%],Joe[35%]
49		⊟ Closing	88 hrs	15 days	Fri 9/19/03	Thu 10/9/03	0%		
50		Procurement Audit	20 hrs	5 days	Fri 9/19/03	Thu 9/25/03	0%	30	Sue[25%],Steve[25%]
51		Financial Closure	20 hrs	10 days	Fri 9/26/03	Thu 10/9/03	0%	50	Sally[25%]
52		Lessons Learned	30 hrs	7 days	Fri 9/19/03	Mon 9/29/03	0%	30	Sue[54%]
53		Completion Document	16 hrs	3 days	Tue 9/30/03	Thu 10/2/03	0%	52	Sue[67%]
54		Formal Acceptance (Approval of Completion Document)	2 hrs	1 day	Fri 10/3/03	Fri 10/3/03	0%	53	Steve[25%]
55		Celebration	0 hrs	0 days	Fri 10/3/03	Fri 10/3/03	0%	54	Team

FIGURE 3.4. Sample work plan.

The project manager should ask questions of the team members, who are the subject matter experts for this work, to gather the information necessary to build the plan. What needs to be done to complete this high-level task (subtasks)? How long will it take to do the work (work effort)? Taking into account each team member's schedule, how long will it take to do this (duration)? Is there something that has to occur before being able to do this work (predecessors)? Who will be doing this work (resources)? These questions, or a variation of them, will be asked repeatedly until the project manager has tasks defined to the level necessary. This process is repeated with each high-level activity until the project manager and the project team is comfortable that all activities are properly defined. Once this is done, the entire team should review the work plan so they have a chance to review how their pieces fit in with all of the other's and to validate it that it is correct.

The other method of work plan creation is to bring the entire team together to define the activities required. This is the opposite side of the spectrum of working one on one, as previously discussed. This method allows the entire team to discuss the details of the tasks, such as the work effort, duration, resources, and predecessors. Some members of the team who are only involved in a small portion of the project may find this a waste of their time, and the meeting can last a long time.

One way to do this method involves sticky notes. If the high-level tasks are identified and listed for all to see, each team member would write something that they know has to occur on a sticky note, including the work effort and resource. Once all tasks are identified on individual sticky notes, the project manager facilitates putting each of them where they belong under the appropriate high-level task. Through team discussion, each task is placed in the right place. Predecessors are found when the tasks are put in order, one before or after another. This allows the team members to brainstorm on what tasks are needed before requiring them to put them in the right place on the plan. The project manager will document the results into a work plan. A follow-up meeting with the project team is used to refine the details of each task (Table 3.1).

Each project manager should find the method that works best for them to complete the initial work plan. The work plan includes specific tasks that need to be performed to complete the project, and it serves to identify the interactivity and dependencies between tasks. The knowledge of the subject matter experts, as well as the historical information from previous projects, are used to help

TABLE 3.1. Approaches to developing a work plan.

Approach	Description
Guidelines	Approach is according to organizationally defined methodology
Analogy	Approach that uses historical information
Bottom up	Approach identifies specific detailed tasks first and then organizes them
Mind mapping	Approach uses nonlinear or visual method

produce the estimates for the tasks. The work plan is used throughout the rest of the project to understand the status of the project, to proactively plan for the next group of activities to be done, and to gauge the impact of any requested changes.

A network diagram shows activity sequencing and relationships. A sample network diagram can be found in Figure 3.5. In this diagram, the arrows represent the activities with duration in days. The diagram represents relationships and the order in which the tasks need to be accomplished. For example, task A has to be completed before task D can begin. Task H cannot begin until tasks D and E are completed. The path through the work plan that determines the earliest time point at which the project can be completed is called the critical path. This is the series of tasks that, when completed on time, sequentially and without delay, completes all work in the shortest amount of time. In the example below, the critical path is path 2, which follows tasks C, G, I, and J. These tasks are on the critical path, and any delay in these tasks will impact the duration of the project.

Project management tools such as Microsoft Project offer an automated method to assist in creation of the work plan. These tools also have multiple views of the tasks in the work plan, such as the network diagram. Although an organization with a mature project management office might utilize full functionality of these tools, most organizations only use a small portion to plan and manage projects.

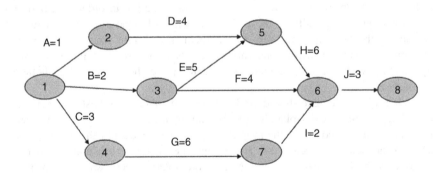

Path 1:	A-D-H-J	Length = 1+4+6+3 = 14 days
Path 2:	B-E-H-J	Length = 2+5+6+3 = 16 days
Path 3:	B-F-J	Length = 2+4+3 = 9 days
Path 4	C-G-I-J	Length = 3+6+2+3 = 14 days

FIGURE 3.5. Network diagram (Schwalbe, 2006).

Time and Cost

Project time estimation is part of the work plan development. The number of tasks, along with their durations and interdependencies, feed into the estimated time to complete the project. Time is the one variable that has the least amount of flexibility. Often, there is a limited budget for the project, which is based on the initial time frame and cost estimates. Decisions and actions made in one area often affect other areas, and possibly other projects. It is important to manage these interactions, as they relate to the triple constraint of time, cost, and scope

The tasks identified and how long they will take to accomplish, plus the interdependencies between tasks feed into the estimated time to complete the project. Identified constraints will impact the time estimate, as well as the critical path. Constraints impacting the time estimate may be in the form of limited human resources, the need for application training before configuration tasks, a limited budget, or required completion date. Assumptions and risks may also impact the time estimate, and each should be reviewed for how they will affect the project.

Cost estimates should include all project costs. Most estimates only identify the cost of purchasing the software application or the necessary hardware, such as servers and workstations. Total project costs should include all expenditures necessary to accomplish the project such as interfaces, team member training, or end user training material development. The most often forgotten cost related to projects is the cost of human resources.

The cost of human resources includes the cost of each employee involved in the project multiplied by the total number of hours they will work on the project. If the work plan includes details such as the work effort, or actual number of hours spent on each task, and the resources for each task, this effort is made easier. Several organizations do not include the cost of human resources because they feel they are paying for their time anyway. It is important to determine if your organization expects this cost as part of the total project costs. Even if your organization does not include human resource costs, they probably include the cost of hiring contractors to enhance the project team.

Some organizations have a separate department that manages the project budget. The project manager should be involved in cost management to ensure the project is completed within the approved budget. There are several tools used

TABLE 3.2. Cost estimation tools.

Tool	Description
Top down estimates	Using previous projects to help estimate costs
Bottom up estimates	Evaluating each individual task or activity to estimate costs
Parametric modeling	A mathematical model to estimate costs
Constructive cost model	Projecting a cost for each line of code written
Computerized tools	Specific applications to help improve the accuracy of the estimation

to estimate budgets. Most organizations already use a specific method or tool to estimate costs. The project manager should check to see which method their organization uses. *See* Table 3.2.

Risk Management

A project risk is a certainty that can have a negative or positive effect on meeting project objectives. There is an art and a science in identifying, analyzing, listing mitigation strategies, and responding to the risk throughout the project. If the project manager manages the risks well, it may go unnoticed by the stakeholders.

The risk management plan documents how risks will be identified and managed throughout the project. This plan should be a standing plan that is followed consistently for all projects. Once risks are identified and documented, along with their mitigation strategies, they need to be monitored throughout the project. New risks may be identified later in the project and should go through the same analysis and documentation. Risks can be closed if they are resolved or the time of their impact is past. For example, if the risk is related to the delay in hardware delivery, once the hardware has arrived the risk can be closed. This risk is closed whether the hardware was delayed and mitigation steps were taken to resolve or if the hardware was delivered on time.

Some risks are identified in the initiation phase and as the team begins to meet, additional ones may be added. Risks can be identified through review of historical information from previous projects, through staff experience, or through general brainstorming activities. Interviewing stakeholders and reviewing the items listed as assumptions and constraints in the scope document can lead to the identification of additional risks. The early identification of risks helps to anticipate possible outcomes, avoid problems, and reduce cost overruns and schedule slippage.

Once a risk is identified, it is analyzed to determine the probability of appearance and the impact to project. This analysis helps the project manager to prioritize the risk so the higher priority risks are watched more closely. Potential mitigation strategies also need to be identified. The project manager needs to determine what should be done if this risk appears and how the impact to the project can be reduced. In addition, the project manager should determine what can be done to prevent or decrease the chance of the risk appearing. This analysis leads to the identification of mitigation strategies.

Communication

The communication plan is important to inform all stakeholders how, and in what form, communication will be handled during the project. Stakeholders need to be related to their communication needs. This helps clarify what communication is planned, who will do the communicating, to whom, how, and when the communication will take place. It also includes reporting relationships and limits, if any, on who can give direction to whom. Contact information for stakeholders should be documented, as well as their role in the project. This communication involves the exchange of information in formal and informal ways, as well as vertically and horizontally.

The project manager cannot assume that everyone related to the project has the same understanding of terms and vocabulary. Common vocabulary ensures effective communication and understanding. Any disconnect between words and actions may cause confusion and require redefinition of the meanings. Any terms used in the project should be defined to ensure a common understanding. Team members who do not have a technical background may not understand terms or concepts such as prototype, failover, interface, customization, disaster recovery, or the difference between a database and an environment. They could also have a different definition in mind, which could lead to confusion. Nonclinical team members may not understand terms or concepts such as interdisciplinary documentation, computerized physician order entry, or medication administration record. Having a standard definition section in the communication plan helps to ensure the entire project team has a common understanding of terms that will be used throughout the project lifecycle and will help to minimize misunderstandings.

The communication plan also includes details about what type of communication is expected throughout the project. Project information needs to be shared with stakeholders and project team members to be truly effective. Historical information can be used to gather what types of communication are needed for a particular project. Some communication should be standard across all projects, such as communicating the project status, which may be done in several different ways within the same project. The team members need to communicate to the project manager the status of the tasks assigned to them. The project manager needs to communicate the status of the project to the sponsors. If there is a steering committee or an executive committee in the organization, they will probably request the status on a regular basis if the project is important to them. Each of these communication types needs to be documented separately in the communication plan because they are managed differently (Table 3.3).

TABLE 3.3. Sample communication plan.

Who	What	When	How	Responsible
Medical executive committee	Project status	Monthly meetings	Verbal report at meeting	Sponsor
Sponsors	Project status	Weekly	Electronically in a status report	Project manager
Project manager	Project status	Weekly	Verbally at status meetings	Team members

The project manager is the center of all communication. The majority of what a project manager does is related to communication in some form. When the project manager communicates with others, the message needs to be clear and concise. If new terms or concepts are introduced, a brief explanation should be included to ensure understanding. When receiving information from others, it is important to verify that the project manager has received the correct message. Summarizing the information back to the sender is a good method to accomplish this. Asking questions at the end of a presentation or meeting to ensure that everyone understood the important points discussed is one method of verifying the team understood what was communicated.

Other Management Plans

There are several other management plans that are either standard across all projects and only need to be documented once or are included if appropriate to the project. Having a consistent way of managing the scope, schedule, resources, and quality helps to ensure a successful project. A process should be defined regarding how to manage changes to these portions of the project before any changes occur. If the project includes the deployment of hardware or end user training, a plan should be written to document how these tasks will be accomplished.

The scope management plan should be consistently followed for all projects. This plan can also be used to manage project requirements if they are documented for the project. Once the scope, or requirements, is approved, any change to either of them needs to be analyzed and approved before taking any action. This is the only way to control one of the main reasons for schedule or cost overruns, which is often called scope creep. The plan should identify who can submit a change request to ensure there is some level of review before the change is submitted for analysis. The project manager should ensure that enough information is obtained about the request to evaluate the impact of the potential change on the project. The project manager is responsible for analyzing the impact to the project. This is done by meeting with the subject matter experts. For example, if the request is related to an interface between systems, the team member responsible for the interfaces should be consulted. The impact analysis should include how the requested change will impact all parts of the project, such as staffing, costs, work effort, and duration, as well as if it will impact other projects or systems. If additional staff is required and they would need to be pulled from another project, it should be noted in the analysis. Once the analysis of the requested change is complete, it is presented to the sponsors who signed off on the charter or scope document. With the details of the change and the information on how it will impact the project, they can make an educated decision to approve, deny, or defer the requested change to a later date or time. If there are several change requests and there is a constraint on the length of the project, the decision may be made to create a phase 2 to include all the deferred requests. The scope management plan and the templates for requesting and analyzing a change should be consistent for all projects.

The schedule management plan is put into place to manage the project to be on schedule and to control change. A schedule management plan states that progress needs to be measured along the way and that the measures of performance are determined in advance. The plan includes a schedule baseline to measure against during the rest of the project. It also includes how any variances to the schedule will be managed, both unexpected changes, in the form of issues, and expected changes, in the form of risks.

The management of resources is as important as managing cost, time, or scope. Resources need to be planned and managed to avoid problems such as lack of resources. Resource planning starts when the high-level resource needs are identified in the initiation phase. Once the resource needs are identified, the available resources should be reviewed to identify any gaps. Each task on the work plan should have resources identified that help with the identification of exactly who is required, as well as when they will be needed. The plan documents the process of identification of required resources, the process of acquiring the team members to fill the needs, and how gaps will be filled. The project manager should determine if there is an opportunity to borrow staff from elsewhere in the organization to fill the openings or the ability to hire contract staff for this purpose. The portion of this plan that needs to be unique for each project is the identification of specific project roles and responsibilities. Some roles will be consistent across projects, but the person who is in that role may vary between projects. The responsibility of the sponsor is consistent across all projects, but the person identified for this role will probably be different from project to project.

The process required to ensure the project meets the needs identified is documented in the quality management plan. The process of how quality will be measured and controlled is documented in this plan. This process may be consistent across projects at a high level, but the plan may need to be modified for different types of projects. The specifics on quality control for a software implementation project will be different than a project to create a new education program. The plan will define the metrics used to document success of the project, as well as when they will be measured, how often, and by whom.

If the project includes the deployment of any hardware, there needs to be a plan for what, when, how, and by whom the hardware will be deployed. If the project is to implement a new electronic health record (EHR) and includes the deployment of workstations to provide access, this plan will define how this will occur. An analysis of where the workstations will be placed includes what kind of space is available in the area, what kind of access is required, and whether network access is available. The space available and the type of access needed will lead to a decision on the type of workstation to be purchased. The specifics of what type of workstations will be purchased, as well as the quantity, will be needed before any purchase. The plan can also define how the workstations will be configured, when they will be deployed, and by whom. Other hardware should also be included in this plan, such as report printers, label printers, scanners, and carts if mobile workstations are planned.

If the project includes training of end users, a plan to document what type of training is needed, who will receive it, when it will be offered, and who will teach it is created. Specifics such as whether or not the training will be mandatory, how many classes or modules are required, and how long each will be should be part of this plan. One organizational or departmental training plan could be used to document the training strategy for all clinical projects, defining the training options and staffing, might be in place. If this were available, the project training plan would only have to define the specifics to this particular project. If this were not available, the project training plan would need to include all information related to the end user training.

Approval and Kickoff Meeting

The project plan is the term used for all plans or documents created during this phase. The creation of these plans is iterative. A change to one plan may impact one or many other plans, which would need to be reviewed and potentially modified. Once the plans have been finalized, they should be reviewed and approved by the sponsor or sponsors. This step validates the information in the plans and obtains the formal approval to execute the plans and move forward with the rest of the project.

The final activity of the planning phase is the kickoff meeting. This meeting includes all project stakeholders, including sponsors and team members. The goal of the kickoff meeting is to ensure everyone is on the same page before the project moves forward. During this meeting, the project charter, or scope document, and project plan are reviewed for a common understanding. Each document is not reviewed word for word, but key points are presented and questions are answered.

The following key items should be reviewed during this meeting:

- The need or goals and objectives of the project.
- What is in and out of scope, as well as the process to request any changes.
- The assumptions and constraints.
- Any identified risks.
- Team member roles and responsibilities.
- Communication plan.
- Schedule and work plan milestones.
- Any other plans developed, such as the deployment plan, schedule management plan, and/or resource plan.

The kickoff meeting also provides a way to validate that all involved with the project agree with the project plan and its components and the importance of the project. The formality of the meeting is dependent on the size of the project, the level of interest of top management, and the makeup of the team.

The implementation of an EHR may necessitate a more formal kickoff meeting than a project to develop a new educational program. Both are important to the organization, but the EHR kick-off meeting is a more visible project to senior management.

Summary

The time spent on planning is invaluable to ensure a successful project. Project planning will help mitigate the risk of the project taking longer than originally expected by setting realistic expectations and controlling scope creep. The plans developed in the planning phase have a single purpose, which is to clearly identify how each portion of the project will be managed and what will occur if variances arise. Being proactive, instead of reactive, in managing projects helps to mitigate any variances, allowing for more expeditious corrective actions.

4
Execution Phase

Introduction

This phase begins the activities to complete the work that was defined in the initiation and planning phases. During this phase of the project, the project manager is focused on facilitating the team members to complete the actual project work. To accomplish this, project managers often need to work on getting the project staff to function as a team to complete the tasks in the work plan. The project manager needs to use multiple management styles, and will function in many roles during the execution of the project. In addition, further project analysis, and even replanning, may be needed. The execution phase of the project usually takes the most time and resources to complete. This is the work that is commonly thought of as project management.

As previously discussed, a project is defined as a "temporary endeavor undertaken to create a unique product, service, or result" (Lewis, 2003). Every project has a beginning, middle, and end; this chapter discusses the middle of the project, although managing the project often has staff longing for the end or even the beginning of the project. All the plans created during the project planning phase will come into play during the execution phase. The project manager will need to manage the execution of the work using these plans to bring the project to completion on time and on budget.

Execution Phase Definition

To execute the project means to integrate people and other resources to carry out the project plans for the project. Execution is not just about the work getting done, however, it is about how the project is managed. For example, during the planning phase, work teams are often asked what is required to complete a deliverable and to give their suggestions based on previous projects or experience. During the execution phase, however, these deliverables need to be completed. Work effort may or may not have been correctly estimated, so the project manager may need to manage the work plan to determine ways to reschedule work effort or modify the scope or timeline. The project manager works to get the team focused on the

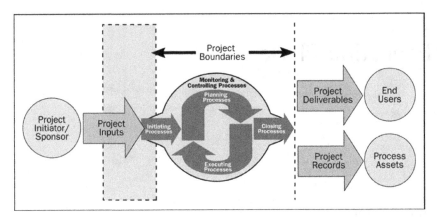

FIGURE 4.1. Project processes (PMBOK, 2004).

work and activities to complete the deliverables defined in the project charter (Figure 4.1).

Managing Project Resources

One of the most important things the project manager must understand is that they cannot sit back and watch the project, and they cannot deliver all the work themselves. The project manager must MANAGE the project and the project team. Although this sounds simple, many healthcare providers do not have the management skills or training, so this is often one of the most difficult roles for a healthcare project manager. It is also difficult because the people on the team the project manager is managing are rarely their direct reports and, in fact, often report to several different managers. When resources are not under the project manager's direct supervision, they often really have two bosses—their direct supervisor and the project manager. Project managers can manage and direct the part of the team members' work effort that falls within the project plan, but not anything else, and there are often conflicts for the team member. To minimize the impact of these conflicts and/or prevent them altogether, the project manager should meet with the team members and supervisors regularly. These meetings should focus on the team members' work and how this work, and any other that the team member is assigned, can be most efficiently accomplished. For example, most projects and supervisors require some kind of status reporting. Sometimes this is verbal, and other times it requires a formal document or record. Where possible, using one standard format to accomplish this will help all the parties involved. Often, for a project, a status report includes work accomplished this period, work planned for next period, and issues/barriers with action plans on the specific project. The specific period, such as weekly, biweekly, or monthly, is often agreed upon in advance. Supervisors, on the other hand, want information on time worked, planned personal time off, career aspirations, and issues/barriers to the employee's performance. One way to accomplish this is to merge both reports into one format. This can allow both the supervisor and the project manager to get a more complete picture of the employee's time and better help them to manage their work efforts. There are times, however, that the supervisor or employee doesn't want the project manager to see any information other than what pertains to the project. Perhaps the project is internal to the department and not for eyes outside the department. Perhaps the team member is reporting on multiple projects and the project manager doesn't want those details shared with other managers. Perhaps the team member needs to report issues with the project manager themselves and how they are working to improve specific project issues. In these cases, the same tools can still be used with some modification. One way is to write the full report and copy only the project-specific details to the project manager in an e-mail or separate document. Another way is to create multiple-page reports that are separated before being submitted.

During the initiation and planning phase, the project manager often works more as a facilitator to gather requirements, define scope, and create the project plans and other deliverables. During the execution phase, however, the project manager needs to use a variety of management styles and skills to complete the deliverables and report progress to a wide variety of stakeholders.

Often, during the execution phase, the full project team meets for the first time. Ideally, the team should meet during the project kickoff meeting, but often, not all members have been assigned to the team and/or changes to the team structure may have occurred. The project manager may have some say in who will be on the team or may have team members assigned to the project. It is important to always manage to the project work plan; i.e., to work to create a team to accomplish the tasks of the project. Team members often come from a variety of departments and/or specialties, and thus report to different managers. Team members come with different work styles and reporting structures, so they need to be managed differently. Sometimes team members don't even want to be part of the team. Team members need time to learn how to work with each other and with the project manager to accomplish the tasks in the most efficient manner and produce the best quality work. They may also need some guidance on how to work together. This is often one of the most difficult roles for the project manager.

Forming Teams

The first thing a team needs to do is figure out how to become a team. One of the most well-established models for team development is Bruce Tuckman's model. (Tuckman, 2005) In his model, which he published in 1965, he describes the phases of team building as forming, storming, norming, and performing. Tuckman's model shows that team members need to mature as a team, and that the project manager's style needs to change as the team grows (Table 4.1).

TABLE 4.1. Tuckman's team development model.

Team Phase	Leadership Style
Forming	Directive
Storming	Persuasive
Norming	Participative
Performing	Delegative

Team-Forming Phase

During the first phase of team building, called the forming phase, team members are learning about each other and how others on the team work, both in style and execution. Tuckman suggests that the best management style for this phase is directive. The team is looking for the project manager to give them structure, a sense of direction to get them started. Starting with meeting ground rules is one way to set up future meetings. Ground rules are intended to help manage meetings and make them more efficient. These include starting and ending on time, having agendas for all meeting, and minutes with action items for follow up after meetings. Other meeting ground rules that help team members show respect for each other include things like silencing cell phones, listening to all team members with no side conversations, and showing up to the meetings on time (Table 4.2).

Starting the first team meeting with an icebreaker exercise can help team members get to know each other's style better. An icebreaker is intended to be a quick way to get team members to get to know each other and be more comfortable with the work. Icebreakers can be informal, such as asking everyone to introduce themselves and share one detail about their work background. Or, icebreakers can be more structured and can include games, role playing, imagery, or sharing. The project manager can facilitate the icebreaker or act as a participant so the team can also get to know them better. If the project

TABLE 4.2. Meeting ground rules.

Start and end on time

Every idea is worth listening to; everyone should contribute and everyone's contributions are to be respected

Create an agenda for every meeting and stick to the agenda

Use a Parking Lot to capture issues out of scope for the current meeting's discussion

No sidebar conversations

Turn cell phones and pagers off or to vibrate

Consensus is used for decision-making as much as possible; otherwise, the 80:20 rule will apply

The project manager has permission to manage the discussion, including time-boxing and redirection manager participates, an independent person should be brought in to facilitate. If the project manager functions as facilitator, they should watch how the other team members interact during the exercise. This will help the project manager learn about how the team members think and how they may work with others. Often, there are team members who do not like to play games, but they should be expected to participate like all of the other team members. Sharing the purpose and the outcomes with these team members may increase their willingness to participate (Table 4.3).

If possible, have the first work meeting in a more informal setting, such as over food at a team dinner. This can encourage team members to interact more naturally. Team members may feel better able to contribute in a relaxed

TABLE 4.3. Examples of icebreakers.

Name	Purpose	Directions
I've done something you haven't done	Help team members get to know other team members and what's important to them. This can be a short icebreaker if people have varied backgrounds.	Have each person introduce himself or herself and then state something they have done that they think no one else in the class has done. It can work related or personal. Some examples include, have 6 siblings, went parasailing, implemented more than 10 applications, etc. If someone else has also done it, the person must state something else until he/she finds something that no one else has done
Famous person	Help team members interact with others.	People write a famous name on a piece of paper and pin it on someone else's back. Person tries to guess what name is pinned on his/her by asking others around the room yes or no questions. Variation: use famous place instead of famous person
Find someone	Encourages team members to intact with others	Each person writes on a blank index card one to three statements, such as favorite color, interest, hobby, or vacations. Pass out cards so everyone gets someone else's card. Have that person find the person with their card and introduce themselves
Dream vacation -	Gets team members to talk to one other member of the team.	Ask participants to introduce themselves and describe details of the ideal, perfect dream vacation

(Continued)

TABLE 4.3. (**Continued**)

Name	Purpose	Directions
Say cheese, please -	Helps team members to identify with other team members. This works especially well with team members who are not attending in person.	As each participant arrives, take their picture with a Polaroid type camera (or digital if remote) and hang their photo on a piece of easel paper in the entrance area of the meeting room in groups of two or three photos (depending on size of meeting - you may have only 2 per group or more if the group is large). Use your creativity and decorate the easel paper to extend a warm welcome and set the tone of the meeting. Once all participants have arrived, ask them to find their partners from the photo display on the easel and spend about 5–10 minutes getting to know the persons. Then have them introduce their partners to the rest of the group and share something they discovered they have in common.

atmosphere than in a fast-paced meeting. Taking a little time in the beginning to start forming the group into a team goes a long way in a complicated project.

Communication

During the execution phase, the project manager, along with the team, will further define the communication methods created during the planning phase and begin to use the project tools to accomplish the work according to the plans prepared in the planning phase. Work may begin slowly as each team member becomes familiar with the work and the team's work methods. This time needs to be included when the detailed work plan is created. Consistent direction and follow through are important skills the project manager must demonstrate. For example, the project manager should establish a method for status reporting that includes all the pertinent information that is needed to manage the project and to communicate project status to the stakeholders and sponsors. Status reports should focus on four questions:

- Are the scheduled tasks completed (in progress) on time?
- If not, what do you need to complete them on time?
- What tasks will be worked on next and do you have what you need to begin them?
- Are there any issues interfering with task completion?

Status reports should be delivered to all stakeholders, including the project team, on a regular basis as defined in the communications plan. The frequency is dependent on the type and duration of the project, but should be monthly at a minimum. Status reports should focus on milestone progress and include an action plan to minimize or resolve issues and risks. Using a stoplight format is often helpful to focus stakeholders on the issues they need to address. Use red for example, for items where a milestone is missed, financial targets are greater than 20% behind, and/or a critical path is delayed. Use yellow to show that progress is in jeopardy because other tasks are delayed, over target, or are 5-15% below or over target, and/or performance indicators are below baseline (often includes items identified by the quality assurance assessment). Use green to indicate that the milestones are all on target and general targets are less than 5% behind or over (Table 4.4).

Solicit input for your status reports from all team members and use a similar process for team or status meeting agendas. Executives overseeing the project often use stoplight icons to give reports to their management (Figures 4.2 and 4.3).

Convening regular status meetings is also important during the forming phase of the project. Status meetings should initially include all team members so that each team member can get to know the process and continue to get to know each other better. Once established, however, only team leaders (if used) should report at status meetings, although all members can be invited. This keeps the meetings to a minimum for those responsible for completing the tasks.

Creating an agenda that flows directly from the project manager's status report will greatly help the project manager to report to their stakeholders. Project managers should use the work plan with milestones to determine the agenda of each status meeting, focusing on currently scheduled work and the next set of work tasks to be completed. The agenda should also include a review of the issues log and any action items from the last meeting. If status meetings are weekly, the agenda should start with the status of any work schedule to start or be completed within the next week. If they are monthly, then focus on the work scheduled to start or be completed within the next month (Figure 4.4).

Status reports and meetings focus on the status of the following:

- Work schedule to be completed since the last status report.
- Work scheduled to start between now and the next status report.
- Issues affecting current work tasks.

TABLE 4.4. Stoplight style status report.

Green	• Milestones are on target
	• Targets are less than 5% behind or over
Yellow	• Other tasks delay may delay this task
	• Targets are 5 – 15% over target
	• Performance indicators are below baseline
Red	• Milestone missed
	• Financial targets are greater than 20% behind
	• Critical path is delayed

Initiative	Criteria	Comment	Follow-Up
Physician Services	●	Missed October realization by $21,000 – Physician services. October financial statements not available until Dec. 8.	Financial statements required for validation.
Ancillary Support	●	Missed October realization by $9,000.	Alternative to offset loss savings needs to be reviewed by sponsor group.
Behavioral	●	Missed October realization by $45,000.	Analysis required to determine if savings in regular hours and increased revenue on South 1 will offset at-risk dollars.
CMI	●	$52,956 lost revenue in October due to lower-than-projected CMI.	
Human Resources	●	Lack of monitoring process for PTO. Negative severance budget for November will be partly offset by positive budget in October. Projected budget to be neutral by end of December.	Monitoring process required for validation.
Clinics	●	Missed October realization by $29,000.	Alternative to offset missed dollars needs to be reviewed by sponsor group.
Finance/Administration	●	Missed October realization by $58,000.	Validation of missed dollars in process.
Real Estate	◐	Two missed milestones: Summary protocols not completed & MMC building occupancy and department space allocation matrix not completed - $1,330,000 at risk.	Initiative is dependent on reconfiguration decision.
Energy Efficiency	◐	Missed milestone: delivery of energy audit report of system not complete – $340,000 at risk.	Initiative is dependent on reconfiguration decision.
Patient Care	◐	Missed milestone: hiring of RNs to replace overtime and agency usage – $31,715 at risk.	Analysis in progress to determine if savings in regular hours is comparable to additional costs in agency and overtime.
Ancillary Clinical	●	On track.	
Revenue Cycle	◐	House physician billing – intervention required from medical directors for remaining malpractice issues.	

DASHBOARD CRITERIA

RED – One milestone missed and/or > 20% behind financial targets; or status report not received.

YELLOW – Zero milestones missed or progress in jeopardy due to red light in other initiative and/or 5-15%; behind financial targets, or performance indicator below baseline period.

GREEN – Zero milestones missed and <5% behind financial targets.

FIGURE 4.2. Stoplight status report (Urbanic, 2004).

Initiative	Overall Status	Unresolved Risks	Unresolved Issues	Progress to Work Plan	Deliverables
Overall Project: Transformation	☀	☀	☀	☀	☀
Accelerated Design	☀	☀	☀	☀	☀
Clinical Documentation	☀	☀	☀	☀	☀
Orders	☀	☀	☀	☀	☀

Key: ☀ GREEN = on time, on budget, no major issues

▽ YELLOW = minor variances or moderate level of risk currently under control that require project team action and project management awareness

■ **ORANGE = major variances from plan, high risk or issues that require immediate project management action and governance awareness**

◐ **RED = major variances from plan, high risks or issues that require immediate project governance or executive management action**

FIGURE 4.3. Project executive summary example.

Purpose: Status Meeting Agenda - Sample
Date:
Time:
Location:
Facilitator:

Invited:	Attended?	Invited:	Attended?

Topics

Action Items	Responsible Parties

FIGURE 4.4. Status meeting agenda template.

- Any risks that require mitigation activities.
- Action plans for any issues.
- Next milestones/steps in the project.
- General announcements from the project manager that may affect the project (information about other projects, from stakeholders, etc).

When team members report on the work scheduled to be completed, they should be prepared to report on the status of any part of the project that they are working on, but focus only on the work that they are currently working on. Have the team member report on progress of the tasks and where they are in the process, i.e., completed, on schedule, behind schedule, etc. If the work is behind schedule, then the team member should be able to describe the reasons for the delay, as well as suggestions to help get the work back on schedule. Once all current work has been discussed and action plans defined, discussion about what tasks are scheduled next should be addressed (Figure 4.5).

Storming Phase

The next phase in team building is known as the storming phase. Team members not yet comfortable with each other and the style of the project manager often have conflicts while testing the waters. During this phase, the project manager

---

STATUS REPORT - SAMPLE

TO: PROJECT DIRECTOR
FROM: PROJECT MANAGER
SUBJECT: STATUS REPORT
CC   PROJECT TEAM, MANAGER
DATE:

Actions/Tasks Completed

•

Next Steps

•

Late Tasks: -

Task Task Name		Start Date	Finish Date	% Complete

Tasks Scheduled to be completed this month

Task Task Name		Start Date	Finish Date	% Complete

Tasks Scheduled to start next

Task ID	Task Name	Start Date	Finish Date	% Complete

Issues/Action Plans

• (include any issues or action plans)

Logistics

• (include any team member time off, etc. in this section)

FIGURE 4.5. Sample status report template.

should use persuasion as a leadership style. This will help the team to understand that they are working in the right direction, that they are a value to the team, and that the project can be completed. Members need some careful managing during this phase, and the project manager will need to plan for the time it takes to address and reassure each of the team members. If the project manager manages well, this stage does not last long and team members begin to show their strengths. During the storming phase, the project manager needs to help all the team members focus on the project, not their concerns about each other. This is key to getting the project done on time, on budget, and with good quality. Team members will get refocused on the deliverables and the project work, and the conflicts will be managed.

Issue Management

As the team begins the work in earnest, project issues may be identified. For example, expected tasks may require additional time or resources, or may not work as initially identified. As team members identify project issues, they should either be resolved immediately or entered into an issue log and prioritized to prevent project delays. An action plan for resolving these issues also should be documented. Some issues that arise may have been identified as risks during the creation of the risk plan. These should already have action plans identified to help mitigate the impact on the project with quick resolution. Risks are known potential issues that we can plan for with predefined resolution plans.

Issue logs should be started with the first identified issue after the project kickoff to capture all issues, regardless of type and urgency. This way, issues that are smaller or only potentially a problem when they are brought up or discovered can be managed before they hinder project execution. Several sophisticated software applications can be used to create and maintain issue logs. Ideally, these logs should allow access to multiple users and reporting capability. Healthcare IT departments usually already have some application they use to manage issues, often via the help desk. These can be set up to help manage the specific issues of the new project as well. Any project issues, however, have to be maintained separately from the ongoing departmental issues so that they can be measured as part of the new project work.

The facility does not need to purchase or use complicated applications for issue logs. A simple spreadsheet (such as Microsoft Excel) or database (such as Microsoft Access), or even a table in a word processor (such as Microsoft Word), can be used successfully for most healthcare projects (Figure 4.6).

Issue logs should collect and maintain general information including, but not limited to, the following:

- Issue tracking number or ticket number: a unique number that is not reused when issue is closed/resolved.
- Short description of the issue.
- Updates as the issue progresses to resolution; should include date of each entry to follow progress.
- Date the issue was identified.
- Expected resolution date; for example, if an issue needs to be resolved before moving to another part of the project.
- Responsible team member.
- Status, i.e., opened, in progress, closed, resolved, etc.
- Action (expected or taken).
- Expected consequences if action is not taken.
- Change request ticket number if generated.

All issues should be reviewed regularly at team meetings.

ABC Hospital Issues Log						
Ticket #	ISSUE	Description/ Plan for Follow-up	Date/Updates	Owner	Open Date	Update Date
	OPEN					
	READY FOR TESTING					
	POST-LIVE					
	MONITOR					
	RESOLVED					

FIGURE 4.6. Issue log template.

Norming Phase

The third phase of team building is called the norming phase. During this phase, the team starts to become more like a team than a group of individuals. They begin to work together and cooperate with each other and the project starts to be the focus of the work. Project managers should adopt a participative style of leadership, to share decisions with the team and empower each member to focus on the work in their area.

During the norming phase, the team continues to work on the tasks defined in the work plan. As the team gets more comfortable working together, the project manager often needs to focus more on scope control. Remember, scope is defined as the work to be done (PMBOK, 2004). Often, scope control is more difficult as the team members become more comfortable with the work, each other, and the users. As they get a better understanding of the applications and the users' needs, often they want to do as much as possible to help the users to be happy. This, however, can lead to the team doing work that is not defined in the work plan or that is out of scope. This usually starts as something small, such as help with an answer that the user has asked or a discussion of a way to do things better or more easily, and may escalate into an entirely different project. Discussions between team members and users could also lead to user-requested changes to the scope. The project manager's main role is to maintain scope within the defined work plan while still listening to the needs of the users and the team. Team members should be encouraged to submit scope change control requests whenever they see functionality that may improve the efficiencies of the project. The project manager needs to give each of the change requests sufficient time to analyze the impact on the project scope, resources, and milestones. Once the impact on the project is defined, the sponsors will decide if the change is worth the impact or not and approve, deny, or defer the request until a later date.

These questions should be part of every scope change assessment:

- What is the change in scope (in detail)?
- What tasks have to be done (or not done) because of the requested change in scope?
- What is the impact to the project duration and the project resources (human and nonhuman)?
- What impact does this request have on other projects or other work being done?
- What is the expected cost, if any, of this change (additional hardware, software, human resources, etc.)?

Often, the analysis time required is in itself a scope change, but time for these assessments should have been built in when the initial project plan was created. Often, project managers add a task that spans the length of the project to cover the analysis, issue resolution, and general team management. Once the analysis of the requested scope change is completed, the project manager should present the change with recommendations to the sponsors for approval, following the change control process. The decisions about what changes to approve will depend on the project constraints and priorities related to the triple constraint; if impact to project duration and timing is a constraint, defer, if impact to costs and budget is a constraint, defer, etc. If the change is small enough to be absorbed into the project without any change to milestones or resources (time or budget), then it should be added to the plan. Any change that is deemed necessary to the project's success that will impact resources, but not milestones, can also be added to the plan if you have the budget to add the resources. Any change deemed necessary, but that affects project milestones (and therefore both time and budget), however, requires full replanning and changes in the timelines and budgets, as well as approval from all the stakeholders as per the change management plan. Major application changes like these can also be added as a future phase to a project to maintain the original project budget and timelines. If these changes are moved to a future phase, however, they should be treated as a new project. It is also very important that these future phases follow the project management methodology with a separate scope, and with project plans to be completed as defined when the sponsors deferred the change. Users are promised things in future phases, but the projects often never get done because of other priorities.

Performing Phase

Finally, the team progresses to the performing stage. Project managers should use a delegative style during this phase. Team members are delivering the work and communicating with each other, and the deliverables are being completed. The project manager can concentrate on analysis of the work, planning for the rest of the project, and communicating progress to stakeholders. This does not, however, mean that the project manager can ignore the team and/or depend on them to complete the task without leadership. It is very possible that the team can revert to the storming phase when issues develop. Close monitoring of the progress and overall team interaction is necessary for the rest of the project.

Quality Control

During the execution phase, quality assurance assessments should be performed. Specific quality control measures need to be put in place based on the type of project you are delivering. For example, in a software implementation project, a quality assurance assessment could focus on the percentage of build to requirements, the status of change orders in relation to overall project timeline, or the quality of all deliverables. If quality is not being maintained, corrective action procedures need to be put in place. This may also require replanning and/or replacing team members who are not performing to standard.

The project manager needs to document and monitor the team's progress. There are several tools available to help you through this phase. The first is the communication plan. This plan is developed during the planning phase, but is used extensively through the execution phase. Keeping all the stakeholders informed of the project and its status is key to the project's success.

Summary

Once the plan is developed, the project manager needs to keep the project on track. In this chapter, we discussed the following:

- Managing according to the project plan
- Communicating regularly with the team
- Phases of team building
- Issues log
- Status report
- Status meeting agenda
- Status meeting minutes.

The execution phase is the phase where the actual work takes place. The project manager needs to document and monitor the project as the team completes the work defined in the plans. Documenting status is the best way to identify risks and issues, as well as accomplishments, during the project. All stakeholders and team members should receive a copy of the status reports, which can be used to get things done.

Your status meeting should follow a standard format based on the project and what tasks are currently being worked on or planned for. Always review the status of the big tasks, the issues log, the risks, outstanding action items, and any planned next steps.

5
Control Phase

Introduction

As discussed in previous chapters, the project manager has a responsibility to facilitate team activities that are needed to complete the project. This chapter will address monitoring and controlling the project to ensure that the project continues according to the project plan and produces the expected results.

During this phase, the project manager facilitates the project control so that potential problems can be identified in a timely manner and corrective action can be taken. The key benefit of project control is that when project performance is observed and measured regularly, variances to the plan are identified and mitigated to minimize delays or cost overruns. Estimates say that over 80% of healthcare projects fail; one third are never completed, and most are over budget, behind schedule, or go live with reduced scope (Kitzmiller, 2006). The reasons for these failures vary, but project control can help improve on time and on budget delivery of projects. Reviewing project timelines, deliverables, and managing issues before they multiply helps to keep project delays to a minimum. The project is like a journey with many stops, with manageable work streams, interim due dates, and checkpoints. During the control phase, the project manager needs to support the project teams with frequent checks and celebrations of the completion of incremental work efforts. This way, the project manager can respond and adapt the project work as needed. If the project manager sticks to a rigid schedule, while ignoring risks and the team's needs, the project will be a failure. Project planning should include contingency planning to reduce risk and help the project to adapt to changes. Healthcare projects often span years and need to be adapted as resources and regulations, as well as patient populations, change. Project managers need to work with stakeholders to identify the risks of keeping to schedules versus modifying schedules or scope to better meet the organization's need for the project.

Why Projects Fail

Many people have listed the reasons why projects fail. Kitzmiller et al. report there are many reasons why healthcare projects fail. These include the following (Table 5.1):

1. Growing complexity of healthcare organizations' increased data collection requirements.
2. Increased regulatory oversight.
3. Poor communication to and among leadership, stakeholders, and users.
4. Organizational resistance to change.
5. Creeping scope.
6. Lack of project ownership.
7. Shifting organizational priorities.
8. Failure to meet customers needs.

Fretty (2006) also identifies six key signs for the project manager to watch for to prevent failure (Table 5.2).

1. Project manager lack of self-esteem.
2. Team member disconnect from project and its objectives.
3. Lack of proper planning.
4. Inadequate communication plan or one size fits all approach.
5. Reporting focuses on form, rather than substance.
6. Lack of risk mitigation.

Reconfirm the Plan

Minor adjustments to a project are often necessary, but the project manager needs to manage overall scope and be prepared to say no. During each phase of the project, the project manager works with the team to determine the best method to successfully complete the project. During the control phase, it is

TABLE 5.1. Top ten reasons projects fail (Fretty, 2006a).

One	Team's skill sets are inconsistent
Two	Too many requirements to efficiently manage
Three	The requirements management process is overwhelming
Four	Requirements may be complete, but ambiguity still leaves room for developer interpretation
Five	Requirements are not realistic and cannot be implemented as defined
Six	Business professionals focus on simple requirements, not realistic ones
Seven	Requirements are clear to the team, but not to the stakeholders
Eight	Requirements review iterations are too time consuming
Nine	Stakeholders don't mean what they say
Ten	Too much rework in managing traceability

TABLE 5.2. Key activities of control phase.

Reconfirm the plan
Assess performance
Take corrective action
Keep stakeholders informed

especially important to reconfirm the project plan and the expected outcomes with all members of the project team, as well as the stakeholders. At this point in the project, there have often been changes to the original project plan, either through general time frame changes or because of scope changes.

Methods to prevent these situations include the following:

- Using mutually accepted milestones and performance metrics.
- Monitoring the teams for signs of discontent, e.g., feelings about too much work, the wrong work, etc.
- Appointing project champions.
- Openly discussing issues/risks and team problems.
- Limiting the number of decision makers.

Reconfirming the project plan involves meeting regularly with team members to discuss their responsibilities and expectations against the project metrics and timelines. Each team member has been working to complete activities and should also report status, budget updates, and known issues, risks, and concerns, along with any newly identified risks or issues. Each risk and issue should be assessed, and action plans should be identified to mitigate their impact on the project timeline or budget. During these status meetings, the project manager should review with the team the activities or tasks that should have been completed or are to start in the near future to help them stay on task and complete their activities or tasks on time. In addition, the project manager should continuously assess the team member's commitment to the project timeline and estimated work hours. Often, as the project ends, the team members are getting information about future projects and plans, but still need to remain focused on the current project. The project manager needs to continue to help the team remain focused on the current project through regular status meetings and deliverable assessments. Keeping to the planned deliverable dates is the best way the project manager can assist the team to move to new projects and teams.

The project manager should also reconfirm the plan with the stakeholders. Often, stakeholder checkpoint meetings have been part of the execution phase and control phase. The focus during the control phase, however, should be on the expected outcomes, performance metrics, and customer expectations. The project manager should discuss the project plan, expected outcomes, and reconfirm that the project is on track and on budget to meet these expectations. Discussion should also include any scope changes that have been approved and may have changed the overall project and/or deliverables and identify where the project is in relation to completing these additional activities. The project manager should ask the stakeholders for their continued commitment to the project timeline, deliverables, and resources. Stakeholders play a role throughout the project, and during the control phase, they should be doing the most communication to their departments and areas. The communication should help inform others of anticipated changes and assess their area's readiness for change. Stakeholders should assess their department with questions like:

1. Is my area ready for training?
2. Have we done the necessary preparation for the changes that the project will bring?
3. Have preproject metrics been collected and communicated?
4. Do all the staff know of the changes that the project will bring, even if they are not directly affected?

Assess Project Performance

By this phase in the project, team members have been working on project deliverables and reporting status and risks for some time. During the project control phase, the project manager needs to assess team members' performance as part of the project team. Often, this is a difficult task for project managers, as they are skilled at managing the project and activities, but not necessarily the people. In addition, each team member has a human resource manager who already evaluates his or her performance in general. The project manager should provide feedback to the human resources manager related to each team member's performance.

Project management and human resource management principles are different. Project managers evaluate performance in a different way from people managers. Project managers are assessing performance to the plan—the time frames and budget—and determining what the team member needs to successfully accomplish the tasks. Human resource managers are evaluating team members to help motivate them to do better as resources. Human resource management is considered both an art and a science. The art is the ability to help people work more effectively than they would without a manager. The science is the manager's ability to do that. Human resource managers staff, direct, and control personnel (Rowen, 2005). In the staffing functions, human resource managers select, recruit, orient, and train new resources. In addition, human resource managers support their development over time. They direct, motivate, and help resources manage change and conflict, as well as prioritize work from multiple projects. Human resource managers often solicit input from a variety of sources, including the project manager, to assess overall performance of a resource.

The project manager assesses the team member's performance against the projected time frames and estimated work hours. In addition, the project manager is looking for any concerns that the team member may identify that may affect the overall project. In this way, the team member has the opportunity to recommit to the project or ask for additional resources as needed. This recommitment from the team members assists the project manager to further plan for any differences between planned and actual performance. In addition, the project manager can take this time to clarify issues and begin to plan any necessary actions related to potential problems.

Leadership Skills

Project managers need to exhibit leadership skills to successfully manage projects. Tom Peters, a well know leader and author, describes leadership with some well thought out statements. He lists 50 characteristics of leaders, and project managers need these leadership skills to successfully complete projects on time and on budget (Peters, 2005).

You can apply some of Peters' characteristics to project managers. Project managers:

1. are willing to say they don't know.

   a. Project managers use the team as subject matter experts to give input to the project plan and ongoing project risk and change. The project manager is the expert on how to manage projects and does not need to be an expert related to the project deliverables. This way, the project benefits from the expertise of several sources and not just the project manager

2. are talent developers.

   a. Project managers are expected to manage, not do. If project managers try to do the activities required for the project, the project will often run into snags and delays because of conflicts in priorities. To stay focused on all aspects of the project, the project manager needs to manage the project and the team members need to do the activities.

3. are visionaries.

   a. Project managers need to be able to see the big picture, and to work on the current phase of the project while planning the future phases in detail. This will help to ensure all pieces of the project are completed on time and come together as planned at the end of the project. In addition, project managers need to understand where their project fits into the organization's goals and mission.

4. love the mess.

   a. One of the best qualities of a project manager is to be able to drill down into the details of the project and organize the information, timelines, activities, risks, and action plans. Taking a mess, multiple facts, and perceptions, and organizing them into the overall project plan is key to successful project management. Often, during the peak of activity, a project can be viewed as organized chaos, where the project manager keeps the chaos organized and on schedule.

5. do and re-do.

    a. Project managers understand that the project plan is just that—a plan. Starting with a list of tasks and a general start and stop date and working toward a final plan requires a lot of replanning. All plans that are created in the planning phase require reevaluation with each approved change to the project, as well as when risks or issues arise and are mitigated.

6. know when to wait.

    a. Project managers can only manage others to complete the project tasks, not do them for the team. Sometimes, this means waiting until the team can complete their tasks before you can move on to the next task or phase; sometimes this means waiting until you have buy-in from the team or stakeholders to get the activities done in the most efficient way.

7. are optimists.

    a. Project managers need to have optimism throughout all the phase of the project. Often, project managers are the only team member who can see the project successfully to completion because other team members are too deep in their details to see the larger picture. Project managers need to communicate this optimism to the entire team so that they can continue to work on the details and understand the progress that is being made.

8. attend to logistical details.

    a. Project managers need to focus on the details of the project plans—what has been completed and what comes next. Small changes in the project schedule can cause large delays when the work is stacked; that is, when tasks are dependant on other tasks. They can also cause changes to the other plans and the details surrounding implementation, training, and communication, for example. By focusing on the little changes in the scope and schedules, project managers can prevent big delays.

9. make mistakes.

    a. Remember, project managers are human too, and all humans make mistakes. It is most important to own up to mistakes as soon as they are identified, hopefully by the project managers themselves, and immediately identify an action plan to minimize any risks or issues.

10. nurture other leaders.

    a. There are often stars among the team members. Project managers notice these stars. Nurturing these stars to do their best, to grow, and to stretch their skills within the project and beyond, is one of the roles of any manager.

11. network.

   a. Project managers often solicit the help of other project mangers, especially when there are performance issues. Other project managers have probably had the same type of problem and can often recommend an action plan to help rectify the problem. Having access to other project managers is also very useful to help with project templates, documentation, or any other general project questions.

12. master their organizations.

   a. All organizations have their own cultures, policies, tasks, or people that are considered untouchable. An understanding of these things and the general culture are essential to successful project management.

13. enjoy leading.

   a. Often, project managers get their start leading projects because they were good at their job working within a project team. To be a good project manager, however, you need to enjoy leading, guiding, and motivating others to get the work done well, while helping them to grow. If this isn't something that a project manger enjoys, then the team members will sense that and find it hard to follow them as a leader.

14. know themselves.

   a. Understanding what make people tick starts with an understanding of what is important to oneself. To lead others, project mangers need to have a strong understanding of their own motivation, skills, and strengths, as well as attributes they lack.

15. accept responsibility.

   a. Most importantly, project mangers must accept responsibility for their projects: the team members, the project plan, the project scope, and the success or failure of the project.

Project managers are leaders, and having these skills will help the project run more smoothly.

Take Corrective Action

One of the most important roles of the project manager in this phase is to anticipate potential problems, to control changes, and recommend an action plan to prevent delays and cost overruns.

During this phase, the project manager uses all the tools created during previous phases, including the change control, schedule control, quality assurance control, and scope management documents, as well as budget management and preferences (both the people and the project). These plans form the basis for the project manager to manage the project team and performance reporting. In addition, the project manager focuses a lot of time on controlling the schedule and making sure that required activities are being completed on time. Throughout the project, team members report their progress toward completing their activities. The project manager should be comparing their reported progress, or actuals, to the current project plan, and make any necessary modifications that are needed to keep the project on track.

If team members or other resources are not available, the project manager needs to determine what corrective actions are necessary to get the project back on target. If more resources are required, the project manager should formally request the additional resources, type of resources needed, and a detailed explanation of why the request is required. If the project timelines are delayed for any reason, the project manager should describe the reasons and an action plan to get the project back on track.

Keeping People Informed

Stakeholders often require more information as the project is nearing completion. Risk management is also important in this phase because risks seem to be magnified as the project nears its completion. Routine status reports need to continue and are important to keep all informed of the project status and to reassure everyone that the project will be completed on time or when it will end. Use these status reports to highlight performance/the project manager's, the team member's, and the project's. This is the time to begin to focus on getting the project to closure and highlighting a person's performance as the project closes and resources begin to move on to other projects. In addition, highlight any scope changes and how they have affected the project to keep everyone on the same page in relation to project time frames and budget. Identify any action plans that will be used to minimize risks and keep the project on track. Include details about the budget to keep all stakeholders informed and to minimize surprises when they get the final project budget report. Document and track issues, including who is responsible and when they must be done; this will help to avoid any last minute changes to the project timeline. Many folks do not need to manage a budget during a project. If you do, keep it simple. Track the hours people work on the project related to what they were scheduled to work and report it regularly at status meetings and/or other project meetings.

Managing Project Budgets

Project managers are usually responsible for the project budget, both creating it and managing it throughout the project. This is very dependent on the organization. If the project manager is not responsible for creating and managing the budget, they should have some input into creating it and should keep it in mind throughout the project. Budgeting is a part of project management that is especially difficult for healthcare projects because of the way hospitals manage budgets. Budgeting, however, is a necessary part of the project. Budgets can be simple, such as just the hours for the project manager, or more detailed and include multiple teams, departments, and resources. Starting each budget with standard questions or a template will make the process easier and more successful.

Budgets should include:

- Resource hours.
- Hardware costs for end user devices, computers, printers, servers, and any construction needed to support the hardware.
- Software costs, including license and maintenance fees.
- Training costs, including cost of development of materials.
- Travel expenses.
- Third party costs, including subscriptions fees and consultants.
- Live support.
- Contingency budget (such as 10% additional fees for implementation).

Many facilities have a standard budgeting tool, and most can easily be translated into an Excel spreadsheet. To start with a simple budget, create a column for each month of the project. Budgets should be measured and reported at least on a monthly basis, so the reporting mechanism should be set up to support this. After the project manager creates a column for each month of the project, they should then add rows for each major category that will be managed. Before creating the actual entries, the project manager can do some simple estimates on cost. Use an average hourly rate to calculate team costs based on the hours in the work plan. Additionally, in Microsoft Project, the project manager can add an hourly rate and overtime rate to each resource in the tool. This can help estimate the team costs, but will not cover other categories. The budget is often created at high levels during the initiation phase, but is detailed further during the planning phase, and managed during execution and control phases.

Once the categories for the budget are identified, general calculations will help to determine other estimates. In larger projects, a total cost of ownership (TCO) with individual costs and return on investment is often generated as part of the selection or negotiation phases of a project. A TCO will assist the project manager in identifying the categories needed in the budget, as well as a starting point for the totals that were anticipated during the selection phase. These estimates are supported by project assumptions. For example, many facilities estimate end user devices with a ratio of device-to-patient during the negotiation phase. Once the project begins, however, the hardware assessment may change during the planning phase. Project managers should use the TCO as an estimate to the budget, not the final numbers.

Earned Value Management (EVM)

Earned Value Management (EVM) is a project management tool that objectively evaluates project progress and helps to predict future performance trends. Project managers can determine how well a project is meeting scope, time, and cost by comparing actual information to the planned information, or baseline. The baseline is the original work plan plus approved changes to the planned work. Earned value management has been used by the Department of Defense since the 1960s, and today more companies are realizing the value of using this tool to control costs and schedule. It has been accepted by the American National Standards Institute/Electronic Industry Association as a new standard called ANSI/EIA 784.

It provides an early warning of performance problems, while there is time for corrective action. Most organizations who track EVM measurements do so on a monthly basis. This provides the opportunity to monitor project progress and any corrective actions that have been taken to bring the project back on track. Shorter projects are less likely to get off track as compared to longer projects. These measurements can be monitored more frequently, if necessary, for shorter projects or projects in trouble.

Earned value management begins with three calculated values for each activity, or group of activities, from the project's work plan.

Planned value (PV) was previously called budgeted cost of work scheduled. Planned value is the portion of the total estimated costs to be spent on an activity during a given period.

Actual cost (AC) was previously called actual cost of work performed. Actual cost is the total amount spent on a task up to the current date or total direct and indirect costs from work on an activity during a given period.

Earned value (EV) was previously called budgeted cost of work performed. Earned value is the budgeted cost of work completed as of the current date and is based on the planned costs and the rate at which the team is completing the work to date. The rate of performance (RP) is the ratio of actual work completed to the percentage of work planned to have been completed at any given time.

Additional measurements assist with evaluating costs and scheduling of the project, and assist with future performance predictions.

Cost variance (CV) is the difference between the work that has been accomplished (in dollars) and how much was spent to accomplish it, or earned value less the actual cost. If the CV is a negative number, the work cost more than planned. If the CV is a positive number, the work cost less than planned.

Schedule variance (SV) is the difference between what was planned to be completed and what has actually been completed as of the current date, or earned value less the planned value. If the SV is a negative number, the duration of the work was longer than planned. If the SV is a positive number, the duration of the work was shorter than planned.

Cost performance index (CPI) is the ratio of earned value to actual cost. This ratio is used to estimate the projected cost of completing the project. If the CPI equals, 1 the actual costs are equal to the budget. If the CPI is less than 1, the

TABLE 5.3. EVM calculations.

Earned value formulas	
Term	Formula
Earned Value	$EV = PV$ to date $\times$ RP
Cost Variance	$CV = EV - AC$
Schedule Variance	$SV = EV - AC$
Cost Performance Index	$CPI = EV / AC$
Schedule Performance Index	$SPI = EV / PV$
Estimate at Completion	$EAC = BAC / CPI$
	$EAC = EAC - AC$
	$EAC = AC + ((BAC - EV)/CPI)$
Estimated Time to Complete	Original Time Estimate / SPI
To-Complete Performance Index	$TCPI = (BAC - EV) / (BAC - AC)$

actual costs are over budget. If the CPI is greater than 1, the actual costs are under budget.

Schedule performance index (SPI) is the ratio of earned value to planned value. This ratio is used to estimate the projected time to completion of the project. The outcome is similar to the CPI. If the SPI equals 1, the project is on schedule. If the SPI is less than 1, the project is behind schedule. If the SPI is greater than 1 the project is ahead of schedule.

Budget at completion (BAC) represents the approved budget for the individual tasks.

Percentage complete (%Comp.) shows the progress to completion of a task and is related as either earned value/BAC, or simply the physical progress towards completion. If formal earned value measurements are not required, this value is often estimated by the task resource.

To-complete performance index (TCPI) indicates the CPI required throughout the remainder of the project to stay within the stated budget

Estimate at completion (EAC) is a forecast of total costs that will be accrued by project completion based on past cost performance trends (Table 5.3).

Summary

Controlling and monitoring projects help to keep the project plan on time and on budget. In this chapter, we discussed the following:

- Reconfirming the plan
- Assessing team performance
- Leadership skills
- Differences between project and people managers
- Taking corrective action
- Keeping people informed.
- Managing project budgets
- Earned value management.

6
Closing Phase

Introduction

The closing phase is the final phase of the project life cycle. Final verification and validation occurs to ensure that the final product or project outcome meets the objectives outlined in the beginning of the project by the sponsors. Formal acceptance of the project by the sponsors is a key part of completing the project. The deliverables for this phase include verification audit results, lessons learned, end of project performance reporting, and the closure document, which is signed by the sponsors. The formal acceptance states that the sponsors agree that all work has been completed according to the plans made and that they agree the project is complete.

Verification

If anything was purchased for this project (i.e., hardware, software, or contractor services) a final procurement audit should be done. The final procurement audit is a report that summarizes the results at the completion of the project. This audit verifies that what you purchased is what you received and that the product is functioning as expected. Periodic audits should be scheduled throughout the project as hardware/software is delivered and configured or as contractor services are performed. These periodic audits are done as part of the controlling phase. If anything was not as expected, the steps taken to resolve the discrepancies and results should also be described.

The product or service that was described in the scope document also needs to be verified. During the closing phase, the project manger needs to determine if the services meet the needs of the sponsors and the business involved. Each item listed in the scope document, as well as all approved change requests, should be verified to ensure they were met. This verification can be done through user acceptance testing (UAT) or though a formal acceptance period after it is in use. Several questions should be asked as part of this verification step. These questions include the following:

1. Does this final product meet all the requirements documented in the planning phase?
2. Can the users use this product as expected and does it fit into their business process?
3. Does the final product meet the need identified in the initiation phase?
4. Have all the Measures of Success, listed in the scope document, been met?
5. Is the sponsor willing to accept the final product?

If the answer to any of the first four questions is no, then the project manager needs to determine if the product or services are acceptable to the sponsors, and if not, what can be done to make it acceptable. Something may have changed since the project began that ultimately changed some of the decisions made in the beginning. The result of a risk, constraint, or incorrect assumption may have changed the outcome in a manor that is acceptable in the end. These need to be noted and explained in detail as part of the final procurement audit.

The financial status of the project is also verified during the closing phase. This begins with the initial planned budget, which is used as a baseline. All actual expenses are used in the final financial report. Each line item should have a comparison between the budget and actual costs to determine the outcome. If you are on budget, the balance should be $0.00. If you end up over budget, the final balance will be a negative number. A positive number shows that you were able to accomplish the project under budget. As mentioned previously, projects do change during their lifecycle. If the project ends up over budget or under budget, an explanation should be included. Some project budgets include a contingency fund that is in place as a risk mitigation strategy for the risk of going over budget. This is usually in place when the risk of going over budget has a high probability of occurring (Tables 6.1 and 6.2).

TABLE 6.1. Examples of reasons to be over budget.

Approved changes to scope; additions or a change that required additional work
Change in needed skill set that requires higher cost resource
Unforeseen risks
Inaccurate assumptions
Unknown risks or constraints that appear
Task durations or work efforts that were underestimated

TABLE 6.2. Examples of reasons to be under budget.

Approved changes to scope; removed items or a change that required less work
Change in needed skill set that allowed for a lower cost resource
Task durations or work efforts that were overestimated
Estimates included contingency money for risks that did not appear

Lessons Learned

One of the most important tasks in the closing phase is to document the lessons learned from the project. I'll say it again—documenting your lessons learned is one of the most important tasks in the closing phase. This is important enough to repeat, and it cannot be stressed enough. The lessons learned document identifies what went right during the project, as well as areas that need improvement, during a retrospective view of the project. It is used as historical information for future projects to improve planning. All project team members, as well as key stakeholders, should be involved in this process. The project manager facilitates this process and puts the final document together.

This effort can be done in one large meeting or in a series of meetings. The team should be together for this activity because the discussions can provide valuable information. The project manager should come to the meeting prepared with specific questions to facilitate the discussion such as "What went well that helped you do your job?" or "In hindsight, what could we have done differently to make this project better or go smoother?" This is a brainstorming activity, as there are no right or wrong answers. It is important to ensure this does not end up being a finger-pointing exercise. The intent is to document what went right to help future projects. The team should also try to note what could be done differently in future projects to avoid what didn't go well. The project manager needs to keep the team focused on the intent of this exercise rather than focusing on what went wrong.

During the lessons learned meetings, it is helpful to document the "what went right" and the "lessons for next time" so everyone can view during the discussion. This can be done by using flip charts, papers hung on a wall, or online in real time while the group is talking. The project manager should try to focus on one area at a time, usually starting with what went right. Ask questions that focus on what went specifically well that should be done next time. This could include anything from a team that worked well together, clearly defined roles and communication plan, a team involved in development of the work plan, support from administration or business, or the detailed planning for activation.

When asking for the lessons for next time, it is important to keep the group focused on the purpose of identifying the areas for improvement. If something is noted that went badly, ask how it could be improved, as the intent is to learn from what did not go well and not dwell on the problems. It is sometimes very hard to keep the team properly focused during this portion of the meeting. This could include anything from training started too early and staff forgot what they learned, too little time planned for specific tasks, appropriate contingency plans were not in place, inadequate staffing were onsite for the activation, or the potential benefit of a parallel test that was not performed.

The document should have the lessons listed with a general statement followed by some specific details. You could list "Training started too early" as a lesson for next time. The description could include details such as training was started

TABLE 6.3. Project lessons learned.

Project Successes:

Practice of Activation Activities: A dry run or practice upgrade was done when the initial development environment was created. This allowed the team to ensure they knew what to expect and verified the activation checklist and the details listed in it. This should be the standard method of doing upgrades in the future.

Staff Location During Activation: Having all the staff together in one location worked really well, as far as communication and troubleshooting are concerned. There were a few exceptions for those who were required to be in the data center for their tasks or who were away taking a break. Using radios for communication with these team members was critical.

Areas for Improvement:

Training Plan: Not all staff attended training sessions; this needs to be mandatory. The staff that attended the early classes did not remember everything taught; sessions should be run closer to the activation or a method of refreshing the education should be planned.

Postactivation Support: The planning for post-live support should include relief for the staff involved in the activation activities so they have time to rest. There wasn't any coverage plan to relieve application administrators who were onsite throughout the activation activities.

---

10 weeks before the activation and during the hours after activation, it became clear that the staff who attended the initial training had many more questions than those who attended in the weeks closer to project initiation. Additional classes could be added each day to decrease the duration of training. Some examples of lessons learned documentation are listed in Table 6.3.

You will find that not all information noted in the meeting is appropriate for the final document. Some might be too detailed, such as a team member saying "being able to sit next to Jim helped me because we could help each other with troubleshooting" or "I am glad Sara had a radio when she was in the data center when we had the issue that required the server to be rebooted." These could both be included in the item above titled "Staff Location During Activation." When these are brought up, the project manager could try to summarize before documenting on the flipcharts so the team feels their comments are heard and will be included with their intended meaning.

Formal Acceptance

Another important task during the closing phase is obtaining the formal acceptance from the sponsors. This shows that the sponsors accept the final output of the project and agree it is complete. The completion document compares many of the items from the scope document with the outcomes of the project and defines any discrepancies between the two. The sponsors have a chance to add any comments and sign-off their approval and formal acceptance of the end of the project.

As a project progresses through its lifecycle, modifications to the plans occur. No project progresses exactly as originally planned. A single approved change

TABLE 6.4. Project completion: scope.

Project Scope:

- Create a website for end users and technical staff to provide information to the CRIS project team so they can register the workstations. *Done*
- The website will reside on the NIH Intranet. *Done*
- The website will utilize the CRIS template for items such as color, fonts, etc. *Done*
- The website will provide directions for finding Workstation ID on PC or Mac computers. *Done, although it did not include directions for Mac OS9*
- There will be a report listing the workstations to be registered that will print daily and on demand. *Done*
- Link to this website will be available on the CRIS website. *Done*

to the scope can impact every aspect of the project. At the end of the project, it is important to document what actually occurred during the project. This is done by comparing the original plan to the actual activities.

The original documented scope plus any approved changes should be listed. Each should be noted if they were actually accomplished as written or not. If they were not accomplished as written, the reason why should be noted. There should be a scope change for anything removed from scope, but because of limitations, an item that was in-scope might not be completely the same as described in the scope document. The sponsors should already be aware of this, and the variance should be noted (Table 6.4) .

The project milestones should also be noted along with any changes that occurred during the project. This is done by listing the milestones with the estimated completion date and the actual completion date. If these dates are not the same, a brief explanation on why these are different should also be included (Table 6.5) .

This analysis should also be done for the measures of success, assumptions, and constraints, as well as the implementation strategy. Some measures of success will not be able to be evaluated at this time and this should be noted. For example, a 25% increase in physician order entry within 3 months after implementing Computerized Physician Order Entry is defined as a measure of success, but it will not be able to be evaluated until 3 months after activation.

TABLE 6.5. Project completion: milestones.

Milestone	Est. completion date	Actual completion date
Scope document approved	March 1, 2006	March 1, 2006
Requirements complete	March 17, 2006	March 17, 2006
Development complete	April 14, 2006	April 28, 2006
Testing complete	May 5, 2006	May 19, 2006
Training complete	May 18, 2006	May 31, 2006
Activation	May 20, 2006	June 3, 2006

Actual dates were adjusted due to the impact on the schedule of the 3 approved scope changes that took extra work to develop.

The project manager should be able to document the project completion with some assistance from other team members or stakeholders. Once documented, the sponsors that signed the scope document should sign the completion document, signifying that they accept the project. Without this sign-off, the project may not be considered complete.

It is also important to update the risk plan. This plan should include all risks identified during the project, as well as the mitigation strategies planned and undertaken. If any of the risks occurred, the mitigation steps or corrective actions should also be documented. The final risk plan, with this updated documentation, is extremely valuable in planning the next project, as it becomes part of the historical information from this project.

End of Project

Once the documentation is completed, it should be archived for access in the future. This could be accomplished by putting all files on a CD or in a specific location on a shared drive. Key documents should be kept in hard copy in a secure location, as well as electronically. These documents include the scope, requirements (if done) and the completion documents after they are all signed. Suggestions for additional hard copy documents include original and final project plans, lessons learned, and risk documents. Copies of any or all of the plans created for the project could also be kept in hard copy if desired.

One last activity should occur before releasing the project team. The end of any project should be celebrated. This could be something as simple as an email congratulating the team on a good job or as elaborate as a party with food and an award for each member. Typically the size of the celebration is dependent on the size of the project and the available funds. The organization's culture also plays a role in deciding how to celebrate. Each team member should be recognized in some way at the end of the project. The easiest way to do this, as noted above, is to send out a global email thanking everyone for their hard work. The team member's manager should be included when you thank the team for their hard work. Printed certificates of achievement—thanks are inexpensive, but appreciated by most staff. Creative thinking is beneficial, especially if the budget is tight.

Summary

The closing phase is the final phase of the project. The project manager works to ensure the project deliverables are verified and acceptable to the sponsors. All project documentation should be completed and archived before releasing any resources, as they will be involved. Celebrating the end of the project and its success is an important component of this phase, and is the last activity to be carried out.

7
Applying the Project Management Process in Healthcare Informatics

Introduction

The project management process can be applied in many settings. Every business from the National Air and Space Association to medication manufacturing uses some form of project management, and the healthcare industry is no exception. In healthcare facilities, using the project management process should be the norm when implementing software, upgrading systems, or performing ongoing system changes. These are all projects. All the phases of the project management process lend themselves well to successfully completing healthcare informatics projects. Leaders without a clear understanding of the process won't be as successful as those who understand and follow the process while completing projects. This chapter will focus on using the project management process in healthcare informatics.

System Selection Projects

Often, new computer applications begin as a solution to quality assurance or healthcare risk challenges. These challenges could include the need to reduce medication errors by implementing bar code scanning and an electronic medication administration record. Perhaps the project begins with the challenge of creating a plan to get physicians involved in Physician Computer Order Entry. Lengthy accounts receivable days or less than optimal collections could lead to the challenge of selection for a new patient financial system.

All system selections should start with a plan detailing the activities and time frames, as well as the deliverables expected. Often, the stakeholders of a certain group, such as the physicians or the financial department, start by putting together a high-level needs assessment for the application. This needs assessment describes "why" a new system is needed, but usually does not include "how" to select the system. Once the needs assessment is approved, the project manager can begin to create the project plan for the selection project. The project charter/scope document should include both the anticipated high-level activities and the anticipated costs required to complete the plan. Often, this part of the project begins with a project plan that includes an end date, which is often timed in relation to the budget process; for example, complete the selection by the fiscal year end. The high-level tasks for this plan include the following:

- Application scope definition
- Stakeholder/department identification
- Requirements identification
- RFI analysis
- Software demonstrations
- Reference checks
- Site visits
- Cost benefit analysis.

Using the high-level tasks, have a team of stakeholders identify the time frames and subtasks to help determine the completed project plan. This way, the stakeholders will be a part of all the steps of the decision-making processes (Figure 7.1).

One excellent source to help the project manager plan a system selection is Gartner (www.gartner.com). Gartner offers the combined brainpower of more than 1,200 research analysts and consultants who advise executives in 75

ID	Task Name	Duration	Start	Finish
1	**System Selection**	83 days	Wed 9/1/04	Fri 12/24/04
2	Phase 1 - Project Start-up and Vendor Screening	80.25 days	Wed 9/1/04	Wed 12/22/04
3	Initiate Project	11 days	Wed 9/1/04	Wed 9/15/04
16	Project Meetings	80.25 days	Wed 9/1/04	Wed 12/22/04
34	Screen Vendors	26 days	Wed 9/8/04	Wed 10/13/04
42	Vendor Fair	27 days	Wed 9/8/04	Thu 10/14/04
45	Phase 2 - Focus Group Process	68 days	Wed 9/1/04	Fri 12/3/04
46	Conduct Selection Committee Kick-off Meeting	20.25 days	Wed 9/1/04	Wed 10/13/04
52	Develop Demonstration Scripts	39 days	Wed 9/1/04	Mon 10/25/04
67	Prepare for Demonstrations	15 days	Thu 10/14/04	Wed 11/3/04
68	Invite participants	1 day	Thu 10/14/04	Thu 10/14/04
69	Develop demonstration scoring tool	3 wks	Thu 10/14/04	Wed 11/3/04
70	Demonstrations	10 days	Mon 11/8/04	Fri 11/19/04
74	Analyze Demonstration Scoring	3.6 wks	Fri 11/5/04	Fri 12/3/04
75	Review Demonstration Findings	2 hrs	Wed 12/1/04	Wed 12/1/04
76	*Complete Vendor Demonstrations*	*0 days*	*Fri 12/3/04*	*Fri 12/3/04*
77	Phase 3 - Select Vendor Finalists	83 days	Wed 9/1/04	Fri 12/24/04
78	Vendor Reference Checks	13 days	Mon 10/11/04	Wed 10/27/04
84	Vendor Site Visits	13 days	Mon 11/29/04	Wed 12/15/04
88	*Complete vendor reference checks/site visits*	*20 days*	*Wed 9/1/04*	*Tue 9/28/04*
89	Compile all vendor information (RFI responses, demo rankings, si t	5 days	Thu 12/16/04	Wed 12/22/04
90	Review all Findings	1 day	Wed 12/22/04	Wed 12/22/04
91	*Select 1st & 2nd Choice Vendors*	*1 day*	*Thu 12/23/04*	*Thu 12/23/04*
92	Present Vendor of Choice to Steering Committee	1 day	Fri 12/24/04	Fri 12/24/04

FIGURE 7.1. Sample system selection work plan.

countries every day. They publish tens of thousands of pages of original research annually and answer more than 215,000 client questions every year. Gartner was founded in 1979 by technology thinkers who saw the growing need for well-researched, independent advice. Our culture is still based on the diligent work of exceptional thinkers acting together to apply the very latest knowledge rapidly and effectively. More information can be found at their website. In addition, several healthcare technology books describe the tasks of a system selection.

The business requirements of the new system, not the detailed software specifics, but the general goals of the system once it is implemented, are needed to help define the project scope. Often, once users see what systems can do through vendor demonstrations, the applications that are desired and the potential implementation time can greatly increase. Refocusing all the project team and stakeholders on the goals of the project will help focus all the stakeholders, as well as keep the project on time and on budget.

Often, a system selection project does not warrant a specific budget. Some cost estimation, at least a high level, however, is definitely needed. Most facilities will have some system demonstrations during the system selection. Costs for staff time to attend these demonstrations, the food served, and/or the technology needed should be accounted for. In addition, planning for the costs for site visits also helps to determine key stakeholders as those that must see other systems in place versus those that can participate in local reference calls.

The project manager in a system selection is often more a facilitator then a manager. The project manager needs to coordinate all the activities to complete the selection on time. In many facilities, working with the person who can schedule rooms and the needed technology for the vendor demonstrations and schedule attendees takes up a good portion of the project manager's time and effort. After the demonstrations, the project manager is often the person who coordinates the data analysis and reporting the findings.

Another key role for the project manager during the system selection is coordinating schedules between the attendees and the facility hosting the site visits. These visits can require an overnight trip involving hotels and flights, and coordinating schedules between multiple facilities is usually very difficult. Planning for these dates in advance reduces the time it takes to coordinate the schedules of everyone involved. Once all the system selection activities are completed, the project manager needs to facilitate the final deliverables of the system selection. This deliverable can be as simple as a report to the board with a recommendation, or a detailed analysis of the data and the cost benefit analysis. Many stakeholders are not experienced in this kind of reporting and need guidance to pull all the pieces/the scope, the budget, and analysis/together. Documenting this report, as well as the lessons learned, will help the next group that needs to select a system follow a standard process and do their selection more efficiently.

System Implementation Projects

The projects in most organizations that usually have a project manager are system implementations. These projects can be as short as a couple of months or as long as a couple of years. Various team members are also often involved and usually do not all work for the same manager, so a project manager is needed to coordinate the project activities. Using all of the tools described in earlier chapters is imperative during a system implementation project.

System Implementation Initiation Phase

Once the decision is made to purchase a new application, the project manager begins the implementation project initiation phase. The key document during this phase is the project charter. A project charter is the agreement between the organization providing the service and the customer requesting the service and receiving the deliverables. The project charter includes a description of the project, a list of anticipated project team members and their roles and responsibilities in the project, the level of authority for the project manager and the project outcomes. In addition, the project charter includes what is in or out of scope and measures of success with formal signatures for approval and authorization to move ahead with the project.

Overlooking the project charter can lead to problems for the duration of the project. For example, it is important to the success of the project to have all project stakeholders in agreement on the purpose of the project and the benefits the organization expects to achieve once complete. If the organization plans to implement the Physician Computer Order Entry for example, benefits could include:

- improved patient safety, measured by a 10% reduction in medication errors
- improved patient care, measured by a 10% reduced length of stay
- reduction in costs, measured by a 10% reduced cost per day.

Focusing the work throughout the project on the specific project goals outlined in the project charter will help all team members keep on track and focus on the activities that are needed to be done as documented in the work plan. In addition, the goals in the project charter help to reduce scope creep. Often, when the project team members are working on the details of a project, they see things that need to change and do not realize that working on these items can be outside of scope.

Project charters also define roles and responsibilities, as well as the scope and the project manager's level of authority. If it is a small project and only the project manager is focused full time on the project, the roles and responsibilities clarify the role each team member has related to this project and gives the project manager the authority needed to manage resources in an effort to remain on time and on budget. If it is a large project, which often has multiple project sponsors, the project charter will help focus the work and identify the chain of command.

System Implementation Planning Phase

Once the initiation phase is completed, the project manager needs to focus on planning the work to be done. Because planning is the most important step in the project, longer projects require more planning than shorter ones, so the time must be scheduled appropriately. Many facilities have a planned go-live date that is based on the sponsor's expectations after the system is selected. It is often easiest to plan the project backwards from this selected date. Once you identify the high-level tasks, if the identified date is still achievable, bring the high-level plan to your team members for their input and additional details. If this selected date does not work at this point, use your high-level plan to discuss the triple constraint/time, cost (resources), and scope/with the sponsors to identify a more realistic go-live date. At times, the project manager will need to further detail the work plan to change the original go-live date and/or detail the risks associated with the initially selected date.

Other key tasks in the planning phase include organizing agendas, status reports, and files so that the standards are established for all team meetings and deliverables. Keeping tools standardized makes it much easier as the project proceeds, especially for team members who report to various managers. Using standardized tools allows the project manager to more easily report to the stakeholders, as well as identify any potential problems more quickly (Figure 7.2).

During the project-planning phase, the project manager also needs to create standards or use existing standards for reporting the budget, risks, and any changes in the project plan. By creating these standards early in the project, the execution and control phases of the project will run more smoothly.

System Implementation Execution and Control Phases

Once the project is underway, the project manager needs to continue to focus on the entire project plan, managing scope, and the project budget. All the team members will be able to identify their activities via the project work plan. Team members should report regularly, as often as every week, to the project manager regarding the status of their activities on the work plan. Each team member should identify any activities that are delayed or potentially delayed as early as possible. This way, the project manager will know of any issues and will be able to identify any potential risks early. Risk management is a large part of the project manager's work during the execution and control phases. Once a risk is identified, the project manager can begin to work on ways to mitigate or rectify the problem. Referring back to the original project scope will assist in correcting the types of problems that most often occur and refocus the work of the team. At times, however, the project team identifies additional activities that are needed to successfully complete the implementation. When these additional activities are identified, the project manager needs to follow the scope change management process created during the planning phase and make any required modifications to all affected parts of the project plan. Any changes that require

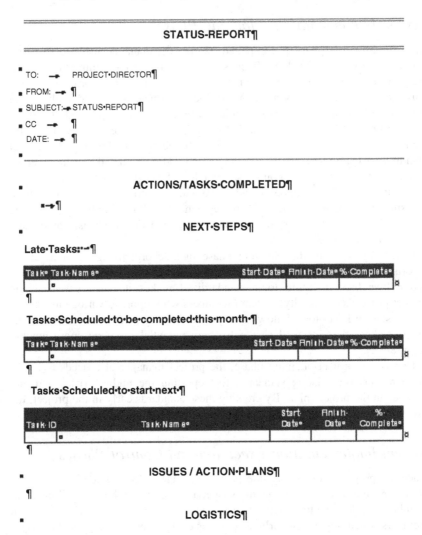

FIGURE 7.2. Sample simple status report.

an increase in time, cost, or resources will probably need to be approved by the stakeholders or steering committee. This kind of change will require replanning of the work plan and, possibly, the project budget.

Project budgets are often the most difficult thing for a new project manager to manage. During an implementation project, the project budget often involves more than just the cost for the human resources involved in the project. The budget can include items such as hardware, training, additional interface work, and/or upgrades to existing applications. These items should be taken into account when planning the initial project, and they may require replanning once the actual costs are identified during the project. Starting with a simple budget plan that can be expanded as the project work plan is completed often helps. Major expenditures that need to be included in an implementation budget include:

- Computer hardware
  - Servers, network, and backup systems
- User devices
  - Point of care, workstations, and printers
- Training
  - Project team training, end user training, training rooms, and training material development and printing
- Project resources
  - Internal, vendor, and third party
- Application costs
  - Initial costs, support costs, data conversion, interfaces, and required third-party applications
- Resource travel
- System or network upgrades
- Third-party subscriptions.

The project manager should plan to include a budget report at least monthly in the project manager status report. Most organizations and vendors have a specific method to report and manage the budget. At a minimum, the project manager should report monthly actual expenditures and compare them to the budgeted expenditures. Any under or over budget expenditures should be explained in the status report. In addition, the project manager should describe how to mitigate any variance in the budget. At times, resources are unable to complete scheduled activities as defined in the project work plan. If this is the reason for the variance in budget, then the project manager needs to identify how the project plan will adjust to this additional work. At times, the work can be moved to the next budget-reporting period, or the work is out of scope and can be applied to the contingency budget, if approved. If the variance cannot be rectified in a future reporting period or by the contingency budget, the project manager needs to request additional funds and readjust the budget or find other ways to reduce the costs. As mentioned in other chapters, if one of the triple constraints—time, cost, or scope—increases, one of the other constraints also needs to change.

Documenting Project Progress

Project managers need to document project progress in a clear and concise manner. Status reports and other project communication should be completed and shared with stakeholders and team members according to the communication plan. Usually, a status report, including a budget update, is done on a monthly basis. If needed, however, the project manager should document any concerns or potential issues as soon as they are identified, and not wait until the monthly status report is due. In some ways, more documentation is better. Using the RACI (responsible, accountable, consulted, and informed) model for reporting is a good way to keep all involved with the project well informed (Table 7.1).

It is a tool that can be used to identify the reporting roles and responsibilities in a project. Coupled with a RACI matrix, it can be a simple, yet powerful, tool for communicating responsibilities, and can be a part of the communication plan (Table 7.2).

To create a RACI matrix, first identify all the activities and list them on the left side of the chart. For a system implementation, these activities can include the major high-level tasks, deliverables, or milestones in the work plan. Then identify all the roles in the project plan across the top of the chart. Once all the roles and activities are identified, the project manager should complete each cell in the matrix. Each activity should have only one responsible role, and each row should have at least one accountable cell. Once the matrix is created, it can be used by all the team members and stakeholders to see where the responsibility and accountability is. This can help the project manager manage the project more efficiently.

Summary

A project is defined as "a temporary endeavor to create a unique project, service, or result" (PMBOK, 2004). The healthcare project manager manages the project from its inception to the completion of deliverables. Job descriptions for project managers often list characteristics such as:

TABLE 7.1. RACI definitions.

Symbol	Definition	Description
R	Responsible	Owns the task/activity
A	Accountable/ Approve	Signs off work before it is completed
C	Consulted	Has information/knowledge about the work
I	Informed	Notified of results

TABLE 7.2. RACI matrix.

	Project manager	Team member	PMO office	Steering committee	Department head	Risk manager
Activity 1		R	A	C		
Activity 2		R	A	C	I	C
Activity 3	RA			C	I	
Activity 4	RA			C	C	I

- excellent communication and strong interpersonal skills
- basic knowledge of computer operations
- ability to use Microsoft Office applications
- interest in the use of technology to improve healthcare practices
- ability to utilize resources
- problem solve independently and work well in an environment with dynamic work requirements
- strong written/verbal presentation skills
- schedule flexibility.

To be a successful project manager, "a leader must acknowledge, embrace and effectively manage various aspects to yield positive results" (Fretty, 2006b). Leadership skills applied to project management help the project manager complete the project plan and activities effectively and efficiently. This chapter discussed two major healthcare informatics projects, system selections and system implementations, where a project manager is needed. By following the project management process, the project manager can successfully assist the healthcare facility in meeting their goals.

8
Applying the Project Management Process in Healthcare Management

Introduction

When project management is mentioned in health care, it usually relates to the implementation of an information technology system. Although this type of project is what brought project management to the healthcare industry, the project management process can be applied to any project. As mentioned in a previous chapter, a project is a temporary endeavor that creates a unique product, service, or result. Healthcare management tackles several projects on a regular basis. The project management process can be applied successfully to complete all healthcare projects. This chapter will focus on using the project management process to help healthcare management.

Project Management Office (PMO) Development

The development of a PMO is a project in itself. The PMO is more than just a group of project managers; it is a methodology for how projects will be managed. It may begin with only one person, or one project manager. The PMO development project is to develop the methodology and project templates for all projects, not necessarily to hire project managers. Understanding the organization's current state is the first step in this project. This is historical information on how projects are managed now and could provide some insights as the project management methodology is defined.

In the initiation stage of the PMO development project, the information gathered should include the need, goals, and objectives of this project. The historical information would include any documentation available from previous projects. Even if lessons learned are not documented, interviewing people who were involved in the projects will help to gather valuable information about what processes should be kept and which ones need improvement. Research on what others do or recommend provides additional information on industry best practices. There are several resources available related to project management in general, as well as specifically for the healthcare industry. The Project Management Institute (www.pmi.org) provides resources related to project management, educational opportunities and resources. Some of these resources are listed in the appendix. All of the information gathered is documented in the project charter or scope document that is created to approve and authorize the project (Figure 8.1).

PMO Development:

Business need

This facility has been unsuccessful in managing projects over the past few years. There is a need for a reusable formal process, using industry best practices, to manage projects of all types. We need to have the appropriately skilled staff to manage these projects.

Goals:

To establish a PMO that will:

- Have a defined process to manage projects.
- Have defined roles and responsibilities for all members of the PMO.
- Provide staff skilled in managing projects.
- Provide mentoring for staff involved in projects.
- Provide ongoing education to staff regarding project management and processes.

Objectives:

- The PMO will have a standard project management process based on industry best practice.
- The PMO will have standard templates for all documents used in the process.
- The PMO will provide education regarding the process to all staff that will be involved in projects before beginning the process.

Deliverables:

- A "Project Management Process" document.
- A "PMO Roles and Responsibilities" document.
- Templates for all documents used in the defined process.
- Education materials for the process and how to use the templates.

Constraints:

- It is necessary to find someone with project management skills to manage this project.
- The staff involved in projects may not accept the new process.

Assumptions:

- The project manager will have the ability to create the PMO and all deliverables.
- The Project Management Institute will be used for reference in creating the PMO.

Relevant Historical Information:

- Documentation from previous projects has been compiled in a single location.
- A list of team members from previous projects is available for interviews related to current project management processes.

Resource Needs:

- A project manager
- A trainer to assist with training materials

FIGURE 8.1. Initiation worksheet.

The planning phase for the PMO development project may include minimal plans for managing the portions of the project, such as risk, scope, schedule, and resources. The goal of this project is to develop these processes and some standardized plans to use across all projects, so they may not be as developed for this project as for future projects. The resources for this project may need to include some contract staff if your organization has limited or no project management experience. This will be determined when the resource needs are identified and compared to the available resources in the organization. The work plan should include work effort, duration, and resources for each item to be developed, each plan, the overall methodology, and roles/responsibilities of the staff working in or supporting the PMO. It is important to start with the basics. It is extremely difficult to go from not having a PMO to having a mature PMO. Start with a methodology that would include the minimum expectations; once this is adopted, the methodology can be expanded. Ongoing education and mentoring is important to set up early in the project (*See* Figure 8.2).

The execution and controlling phases are where the methodology is defined and the standard plans and templates are created. The overall methodology should be defined first. This will direct the team for other activities. Some plans, such as the scope management plan, should be consistent across all projects. Other plans, such as the training plan, might be standard or have a standard template, but would be somewhat unique to each project. These plans will vary, but can be kept standardized to ensure all key items are addressed. Templates for status reports, meeting minutes, project charter, scope, and completion documents should be developed during this time.

Once the entire methodology is documented, and is acceptable to the organization, the PMO development project can move into the closing phase. The project validation and project completion documents should be finalized. In addition, the project manager should document any lessons learned. For a smaller project, the lessons learned can be added to the bottom of the project completion document rather than in a separate document. This allows the sponsors to review all the documents, including the lessons learned, and add any comments or concerns.

Transitioning the work from the project into a functioning PMO is important. All staff who will be involved in projects should be educated to the new process and the expectations. All project team members should be aware of how projects will be managed in the future, as well as how the new methodology will affect them. Staff who will be project managers should receive additional education related to the methodology and how to complete the documents required, as well as some general management education, if necessary. Stakeholders, especially sponsors, should also understand the process and their roles. This should be ongoing, as each new project could have new stakeholders or sponsors. Remember, it is important to have some form of mentoring for new project managers, as well as ongoing education to help fine tune the project manager skills. Brownbag sessions, or lunchtime educational sessions, are a good way to provide additional education.

Tasks
Execution &control
Interview project team members
Review previous project documentation
Resource review for best practices
PMO methodology
Initial draft of methodology
Initial PMO roles & responsibilities
Sponsor review of methodology
Final draft of methodology
Final PMO roles & responsibilities
Methodology approval
PMO standard plans
Scope change management plan
Risk management plan
Resource management plan
Schedule management plan
PMO templates
Scope template
Risk Plan template
Communication plan template
Work plan template
Training plan template
Status report template
Meeting agenda/minutes template
Kick-off presentation template
Scope change request/analysis template
Completion document template
Lessons learned template
Education
Plan for education of all project managers
Plan for education of all project team members
Education material development
Training for project managers
Training for project team members
Schedule for ongoing training

FIGURE 8.2. Tasks to create a PMO.

Interdisciplinary Care Model Implementation

Introducing an interdisciplinary care model to an organization can also be managed as a project. The development of a new process has a defined beginning and end. The transition from a "project" to a "process" occurs once the development is completed, the staff is trained, and the new process is in place and being followed. This transition needs to be defined, planned, and implemented during the project.

The initiation and planning phases are where the current state, or current care model, will be reviewed, and the new model will be defined. The planning for how this new model will be developed and implemented should be defined and added to a work plan. For a project such as this, end user involvement, communication, and education are all important. Buy-in from those affected by the change will be enhanced if they are involved in the process of planning and developing the new model. Depending on how this new model is structured, the project manager needs to evaluate everything that may be necessary for it to be successful. If the new model includes interdisciplinary rounds, for example, will a wireless device be required so the team can view the patient information in real time during the rounds? Planning for hardware procurement, a wireless network, and modifications to the clinical applications might be a required part of the project (Figure 8.3).

The execution and control phases for a project like this should include a user group that can assist with the development and validation of the new process. Modifications to the clinical application to enhance the interdisciplinary rounds may include creating a view or report that provides the necessary patient information to enhance information sharing during the rounds. During these phases, the new model might be piloted in one area of the organization and then rolled out to others in a phased approach. Evaluations after each area is brought

- Current state

  - Meetings with care team user group
  - Document current care process
  - Gather copies of current documentation forms

- Future state

  - Meetings with care team user group
  - Document future care process
  - Modify documentation forms as needed
  - Evaluation of need for new hardware

- Hardware implementation

  - Evaluation of network
  - Update network as needed
  - Procurement of new wireless devices
  - Deployment of wireless devices ahead of rollout

- Future state implementation

  - Configuration changes to clinical application
  - Education on future state for pilot team
  - Pilot test of new process
  - Evaluation of pilot test
  - Modifications to plan as necessary
  - Education of care teams (one area at a time)
  - Rollout to patient care areas (one area at a time)

FIGURE 8.3. Activities to be accomplished for work plan.

"live" should be collected to ensure any issues are resolved before moving to the next area.

The closing phase includes documentation of the validation done during the process rollout. All feedback received, as well as any action taken or planned, should be included in this report. This provides information to all involved about what was done, including the feedback obtained from the end users. It demonstrates that the feedback was received and valued. The project ends when the process has been rolled out to all areas included in the scope of the project. A transition should be made to whoever will evaluate this process in the future to ensure continuous improvement. Documented lessons learned will help with future projects where new processes are implemented. An example of lessons learned from this type of implementation project can be found in Figure 8.4.

New Training Program Development

Developing a new training program is also a project, and it should be managed using the defined project management process. The project begins when the need is identified for the new program and ends when all pieces are in place to offer the program. The outcomes of this type of project include identified courses, training materials, process to register for courses, staffing, and training schedules.

Start with any historical information related to other similar programs at your facility or other facilities that are willing to share information. Professional organizations may also be able to provide some information regarding the new training program needed. The charter or scope document for this type of project should include the objectives of the program, as well as the actual deliverables, such as training materials, that will be produced during the project.

The planning for a training program would include a communication plan that describes how the program will be marketed to the end users. This relates to marketing to those outside your organization if it is an educational program for the community, as well as internal marketing if that is where the target audience is. The work plan should include these marketing activities along with the program development activities. A potential risk for an education program development project could be lack of participation. The mitigation strategy should include analysis of potential reasons why the attendance was limited, such as whether the courses were offered at the time when people were available or was there a lack of interest in the offering. The mitigation strategy should also include what to do if no one signs up to attend the program (Figure 8.5).

As the project moves into the execution and control phases, the development work begins. The course objectives are developed into an actual course offering. Training materials, such as computer-based training (CBT) modules, manuals, handouts, practice exercises, or quick reference guides are developed. If the training includes hands on activities, the tools or objects used will need to be

Purpose

The new Interdisciplinary Care Model was successfully implemented on March 10, 2007. Once the project was completed, the project team met to discuss what went well during the project that should be repeated during future projects. The team also noted areas for improvement that would help future projects be more successful.

Project management and communication
Project successes

- The project management methodology allowed the project to be tracked and organized from beginning to end.
- The user groups provided an effective avenue for communication with end users. This included communication from end users to the project team and from the project team to end users. This only worked because the user group members consistently communicated with the rest of the end user community.
- The use of the "Healthcare Speaks" to communicate the expected changes reached all caregivers. A standing article was in place before, during, and after the deployment to communicate and reinforce the hot topics.
- The change management process for scope and requirements helped to keep the project on track and identify when and why the timeline was impacted.

Areas for improvement

- It would have been beneficial to publish extra issues of this newsletter during the deployment rollout. The regular frequency was not enough; they should have been twice a week during the rollout.
- The change management process should have been followed for all changes to the design, no matter how small they seemed.

Design
Project successes

- The user groups were a tremendous help in defining the current and future care processes.
- Having the future state documented before the evaluation of the network and hardware helped to ensure that the placement of hardware matched the new processes.

Areas for improvement

- Changes to forms need to be approved by the Medical Records committee before putting them in place.

Testing
Project successes

- The pilot test provided very valuable information to make the actual deployment better.
- The information from the pilot test was placed into categories (Activation, FAQ, Training/Communication, and Future Requests). Activation items were all addressed before deployment to the first unit, FAQ were communicated to end users and were posted on the website, and Training/Communication items were added to the training materials and published in the newsletter. Future requests were placed in a database to be evaluated for addition after the entire deployment.

Areas for improvement

- Additional time between the pilot test and the training classes would allow all training materials to be updated before the beginning of classes. Some updates had to be given verbally until all materials were updated. This impacted the first two units in the rollout only.

FIGURE 8.4. Lessons learned.   *(Continued)*

Training
Project successes

- The training materials were created for use in new employee orientation, allowing for an easy transition between the project training and the postactivation training.
- The use of super-users assisted with posttraining questions from end users. Having the super-users from units not live yet spend time on live units kept their skills sharp.

Areas for improvement

- See item under testing regarding the time frame between testing and training
- The training should have been mandatory. There were many questions after activation because not all users attended training. This was modified for units that went live later in the rollout

Deployment
Project successes

- The progressive rollout, one unit at a time, allowed for improvements in the process throughout the deployment
- Tracking all changes during the rollout ensured all changes were made for future and previous units in the rollout.
- Documenting lessons learned from each unit in the rollout allowed for continuous improvement throughout the deployment

Areas for improvement

- The selection of the order of rollout should be evaluated for how the patients and staff move through the hospital. Having patients and staff move from live until to nonlive unit was confusing and caused some impact to documentation during the rollout.

FIGURE 8.4. **(Continued)**

obtained and made ready for the courses. The process for registering for the courses will also need to be put into place.

If the end user will obtain credit for the coursework, the approval for continuing education unit credit (CEU) or continuing medical education (CME) credit will need to be obtained. Many healthcare staff will expect credit for courses they take related to work. Both organizations have a process that needs to be followed to obtain approval to provide credit. This needs to be planned, as the information will have to be sent early enough to receive approval before the course offering.

The closing phase will include validation that everything is in place to offer the new educational program. The project completion document would include information related to the accomplishment of all items identified as in scope. If the scope includes having the first offering of the program completed and course evaluations analyzed, then the project will not be complete until this is done.

Research Project

Although it may be easy to think of a research project as a project, it might not be as easy to see how the process does resemble the project management methodology. Although the terminology may be different, a research project follows the process from initiation through to closure.

Goal: To develop a new training program to provide a prep course for the nursing informatics certification. The course will be offered quarterly.

Project Objectives/Scope:

- Training program objectives:

    - To review the content of the nursing informatics certification exam.
    - To understand the information technology used today, including the solutions used to keep data secure.
    - To understand the process of data transformation.

- CEUs will be provided for attendees.
- Document the day-to-day agenda for the course that will be offered.
- Develop all training materials required.
- The current process for registration will be used for this new program.
- All current trainers certified in nursing informatics, will be prepared to teach the new course.
- Staffing and training schedules will be developed for the first eight weeks of offerings.

Project Justification: The Chief Nursing Officer is encouraging nursing informatics certification with the emergence of more data being stored electronically.

Project Team:

Role	Name	Contact Information
Project Sponsors	Herman Smither	hsmither@xxx.com
Project Manager	Nicole Michaels	nmichaels@xxx.com
Project Team Resources	Joe Vincelli	jvincelli@bbbbbb.net
	Matt Miller	mmiller@xxx.com
	Gary Currie	gcurrie@mmmmm.com
	Marion Houston	mhouston@xxx.com
	Sue Sapelak	ssapelak@xxx.com

Implementation Strategy:
The program will be developed by first defining the objectives and content. The content will be split between the project team members for development of detailed content. CBT and MS PowerPoint presentations will be used along with practice exercises. Joe Vincelli will develop the CBT once content is defined. Once all content and materials are developed, each team member will present their portion of the program to the rest of the team to validate the content and flow of the materials. The trainers will be taught as the education schedule is developed and put into the current training registration process. Marketing materials will be developed by Gary Currie and shared with end users through various methods before the first course being offered.

Training Strategy:
Once the content is validated, all trainers will attend the course. A meeting after the training course will be held to outline key teaching strategies for each section. A key trainer will observe the first class taught by each trainer.

FIGURE 8.5. Scope document.   (*Continued*)

Communication Plan:

Who	What	How	When	Responsible Party
Sponsor	Status Escalated Issues	Email Email/In Person	Weekly As needed	Nicole
PM	Status Issues needing escalation	Email/Status Mtg Email/In Person	Weekly As needed	All team members All team members
PMO	Status	Status Report	Weekly	Nicole
End Users	Training Information	Flyers, Newsletter, email, department meetings	Beginning 6 weeks before start of classes	Gary

Risk Assessment:
Risk – There will be lack of participation, or registered students, for the courses
Mitigation – Analysis of potential reasons for lack of attendance by 1) surveying target audience related to class schedule and course interest 2) post-course survey of attendees related to usability of content in their jobs, if they would recommend course to others, etc. 3) analysis of similar courses offered elsewhere. Contingency plan should be prepared for if no one signs up for course.

Measures of Success:
- Analysis of training evaluations show an average response of 3.5 in a 5 pt scale
- Course are taught with at least 50 % capacity of attendees

Assumptions:
- All current trainers have the knowledge base to teach these courses
- There is a need for this new program within this organization

Constraints:
- There is limited available time in the current training schedule to fit these new courses in. Some current courses may need to be offered less often to find time in the schedule
- There is a limited budget for the creation of training and marketing materials

FIGURE 8.5. (**Continued**)

The initiation phase is where the project is defined and historical information is reviewed. This phase coincides with the documentation of the background for the research and collection of information required for the hypothesis. The hypothesis can be related to the scope statement.

Planning for a research project is as important as planning for any other project. The scope document could include items such as the hypothesis, the methods of collecting the data, the plan for how it will be analyzed and what the researcher will do with the data, and the final deliverable. There are risks, assumptions, and constraints for research that should all be documented. Any risks should be evaluated for an appropriate mitigation strategy. The work plan should include the tasks for collecting the data, analyzing the results, discussion, and a conclusion. The final deliverable of the project would be a paper or presentation (Figure 8.5).

The execution and control phases are where the data is collected and analyzed. The length of this phase depends on the length of the study. It is important to maintain control over the study to ensure that all variables are managed according to the plan and any changes are made only after the impact to the study is evaluated. Risks would need to be controlled as they arise. The progress of the study is evaluated as it moves along the work plan and status reports would be required to the oversight committee or group.

The analysis of the data and conclusion would feed into the final deliverable of a paper, a presentation, or both. This documentation would be similar to the completion document where the original plan (scope document) was compared to what actually occurred during the project. Any gaps from the original plan would be evaluated regarding their impact to the project. This feeds into lessons learned, which is a beneficial exercise for any project and allows for a retrospective review of what went well and what could be done better next time. All of this

		Task Name	Duration	Start	Finish	Predecessors
1		⊟ Initiation	21 days	Mon 1/8/07	Mon 2/5/07	
2		Identification of Need	3 days	Mon 1/8/07	Wed 1/10/07	
3		Background Research	10 days	Thu 1/11/07	Wed 1/24/07	2
4		Documentation of Hypothesis	5 days	Thu 1/25/07	Wed 1/31/07	3
5		Approval	3 days	Thu 2/1/07	Mon 2/5/07	4
6		⊟ Planning	29 days	Tue 2/6/07	Fri 3/16/07	
7		Data Collection Plan	5 days	Tue 2/6/07	Mon 2/12/07	5
8		Data Analysis Plan	5 days	Tue 2/13/07	Mon 2/19/07	7
9		Plan for Research Outcome	5 days	Tue 2/20/07	Mon 2/26/07	8
10		Initial Risk Analysis	5 days	Tue 2/27/07	Mon 3/5/07	9
11		Initial Workplan	3 days	Tue 3/6/07	Thu 3/8/07	10
12		Scope Document	5 days	Tue 3/6/07	Mon 3/12/07	10
13		Approval Scope	3 days	Tue 3/13/07	Thu 3/15/07	12
14		Kick-off Meeting	1 day	Fri 3/16/07	Fri 3/16/07	13
15		⊟ Execution/Control	95 days	Fri 3/16/07	Thu 7/26/07	
16		Risk & Issue Management	85 days	Fri 3/16/07	Thu 7/12/07	13
17		Data Collection	60 days	Fri 3/16/07	Thu 6/7/07	13
18		Data Analysis	25 days	Fri 6/8/07	Thu 7/12/07	17
19		Documentation of Conclusion	10 days	Fri 7/13/07	Thu 7/26/07	18
20		⊟ Completion	26 days	Fri 7/27/07	Fri 8/31/07	
21		Lessons Learned	3 days	Fri 7/27/07	Tue 7/31/07	19
22		Paper Creation	20 days	Wed 8/1/07	Tue 8/28/07	21
23		Paper Submission	3 days	Wed 8/29/07	Fri 8/31/07	22
24		Presentation Abstract Submission	3 days	Wed 8/29/07	Fri 8/31/07	22

FIGURE 8.5. Research work plan.

information could be included in the final paper or presentation. The terminology may be different, but the processes are very similar.

Summary

Managing projects through a consistent methodology improves the chances that they are completed on time and successfully. Often, efforts for non-information technology projects are done when staff has time and are not carefully planned, executed, or managed. They are accomplished during the few moments of free time staff or management has to dedicate to them. These, however, do need to be viewed as projects, authorized as projects, and managed as projects. This will help to ensure they are accomplished within the proper timeframe and that the outcome will meet the goals identified. This chapter discussed a few efforts that would benefit by being managed as projects. By following the project management process, the project manager can successfully assist the healthcare facility meet their goals.

9
Summary

Introduction

The project management process is a methodology that can be applied to any project. A project is a temporary endeavor with defined start and end points. Projects need someone to lead the team from beginning to end to successfully control the triple constraint of cost, scope, and time. Consistent use of a standard methodology for managing projects of all sizes will improve the possibility of a successful project being done on time and on budget.

Project Initiation and Planning

Beginning with the initiation phase, the project manager identifies the project and defines its scope, goals, and objectives. Using a project charter or scope document can help the project manager define his or her responsibility and authority. Sponsor approval of these documents will help focus the organization throughout the project, especially if it is a multiyear project. Healthcare professionals can use the charter or scope document in a variety of project settings. Nurse managers who are implementing a new quality assurance or self-governance program can use the project charter or scope document to define the goals and objectives of the initiative and provide authority to complete the project. The content of these documents help to keep the project team focused on the work to be done. Often, focusing on the project scope and goals helps to deflect blame from individuals when the project gets rough. If everyone involved in the project signs the project charter or scope document, as an agreement on the goals and objectives, they are more likely to follow through with scheduled activities during the project.

Defining the communication plan, risk management plans, and the project work plan during the planning phase will help complete projects on time and on budget. If all stakeholders and team members agree to plans during the planning phase, if the project runs into problems during the execution phase, the agreed upon plans can be implemented. Waiting until there are problems in a project can make it very difficult to get the team and stakeholders to agree on how to fix those problems. Purchasing a new information system, which is often a capital budget item and can include construction or retraining of employees, is certainly a project that can benefit from detailed project planning. Remember that work plans are only estimates of the time and resource effort, so planning is very important to reduce the changes of cost and time overruns.

Different organizations plan differently. Some organizations plan proactively for large projects and include cost estimates for anticipated projects in their strategic budget plans for several years in the future. Healthcare equipment, including information systems, has a finite lifespan, and estimated replacement costs or upgrades can be part of the strategic plan. A project management office (PMO) can help with this planning. Having a PMO with the knowledge of ongoing and upcoming projects, including an estimate of the project time frames and costs, can greatly benefit a healthcare organization. This information can also help slot a project into a time when resources will be available and finances can be allocated or support the need for additional resources.

Execution and Control

Once planned, projects need to be managed through the execution and control phases. Project managers need well-defined leadership skills to support the team as they complete all the activities within scheduled time frames. Closely tracking work completed, resource time, and costs helps to keep the project on schedule by identifying potential problems early in the project. Using the change control and quality assurance process helps to keep all the team members focused on quality deliverables within scope and budget.

Project Management Process

Often, healthcare project managers are not trained in project management methodologies. Instead, they rise through the ranks within their department or organization. This lack of understanding can often cost organizations significantly. People who function in project management roles should be properly trained on the entire project management process, not just how to create work plans. Proper training in project management skills and methodologies help organizations manage projects consistently and with improved success. Project managers using a project management methodology can function more proactively and prevent little problems from becoming showstoppers. Taking responsibility and understanding defined authority is an important part of any project.

Remember, there is no reality, only perception. Project managers help drive the project toward completion only if all team members and stakeholders share similar goals and objectives.

Communication is crucial to any project success. The bigger the project team, the more need there is for communication. Even a one-person project, however, requires communication to stakeholders and sponsors. Even if a project is delayed or over budget, communicating project status can help the stakeholders and sponsor adjust expectations accordingly. Issues should be escalated to the project sponsors as needed for assistance in resolution.

Lewis (2003) reported a study by the Standish Group. This study stated that 86% of all IT projects fail to meet performance, cost, and time and/or scope targets. Of these projects, 33% had to be canceled before completion. Although these measurements were across many industries, healthcare faces its share of project overruns. If the project is successful, the overruns can usually be forgiven. They are not, however, forgotten. Project overruns can delay other projects, force the organization to modify or delay strategic initiatives, and/or cause quality issues. In healthcare, quality issues can lead to a loss in patients, both to other facilities and to error, and a loss in qualified staff, which in turn can lead to other losses or facility closures.

Summary

In today's healthcare organization, some type of project is always taking place. Sometimes projects are small and/or short and have few team members. Examples include implementing a new regulation initiative, holding a job fair, or a major capital purchase such as a positron emission tomography scanner. Some projects are much larger and lengthy. Examples include implementing a new information system, opening a new unit or building, and starting a new clinical program. All of these projects, however, benefit from following the project management process of initiation, planning, execution, control, and closing. When followed, the project management process can help reduce cost overruns, maintain scope, and prevent timelines from slipping. In addition, following the methodology for all projects, big and small, can help with an organization's strategic initiatives and planning. Organizations can better anticipate future needs when a standard methodology is followed, and can base future projects on lessons learned. The project management process and methodologies can help healthcare organizations effectively manage both large and small projects.

Bibliography

Abramovici A. Controlling scope creep. PMI Network. 2000;January: 44–48.

American Nursing Informatics Association. www.ania.org. Accessed April 25, 2007.

American Medical Informatics Association. www.amia.org. Accessed April 25, 2007.

All About Earned Value–Milestones Professional answers the Earned Value questions. www.kidasa.com/information/articles/earnedvalue/index.html

Anderson L, Stafford C. The "Big Bang" implementation: not for the faint of heart. Comput Nurs. 2002;20(1):1–20.

Ball MJ, Hannah KJ, Newbold SQ, Douglas JV, eds. Nursing Informatics: Where Caring and Technology Meet. 3rd edition. New York: Springer; 2000.

Bradford R, Sutton M. From survival to success: it takes more than theory. Nurs Admin Q. 2003;27(2):106–119.

Crawford J, Cabanis-Brewin J, Bigelow D, West J, Wourms R, Pennypacker J. Project Management Roles and Responsibilities. Havertown, PA: Center for Business Practices; 2004.

Earned Value Management–Information on earned value project management for government, industry, and academic users. www.acq.osd.mil/pm

Earned Value Management Part One. http://projectmagazine.com/content/view/46/47. Accessed November 2000.

Englebardt SP, Nelson R. Health Care Informatics: An Interdisciplinary Approach. St. Louis: Mosby; 2002.

Fretty P. Why do projects really fail? PM Network. 2006a;20(3):45–48.

Fretty P. Cultivating culture. Project Management Annual. 2006b;2:11–15.

A Guide to the Project Management Body of Knowledge (PMBOK® Guide). Newton Square: Project Management Institute; 2000.

A Guide to the Project Management Body of Knowledge (PMBOK® Guide). 3rd edition. Newton Square: Project Management Institute; 2004.

Handler T. 2(2003) Steps to take when selecting a new clinical system. www.gartner.com. Accessed July 28, 2007.

Healthcare Information Management Systems Society. http://www.himss.org. Accessed April 15, 2007.

Heerkens GR. Project Management. New York: McGraw-Hill; 2002.

Howe R, Flanagan C. Case managers getting it done: a project management primer. Lipponcott's Case Manag. 2004;9(3):152–159.

Humphrey C. Are you an innovator, a laggard or something in between? Home Healthc Nurse. 2005;23(7):413.

Hunt CH, Sproat SB, and Kitzmiller RR. The Nursing Informatics Implementation Guide. New York: Springer; 2004.

Husting P, Cintron L. Healthcare information systems: education lessons learned. J Nurses Staff Dev. 2003;19(5):249–253.

Isola M, Polikatitis A, Laureto R. Implementation of a project management office (PMO)–experiences from year 1. J Healthc Inf Manag. 2006;20(1):79–87.

Kitzmiller R, Hunt E, Brechenridge S. Adopting Best Practices: Agility moves from software development to healthcare project management. 2006;22(2):75–82.

Koppel R, Metlay JP, Cohen A, Abaluck B, Loclio AR, Kimmel SE, Strom BL. Role of computerized physician order entry systems in facilitating medication errors. JAMA. 2005;293(10):1197–1203.

Lee P, Hirshfield M. Planning with care. Projects@Work. http://www.projectsatwork.com/articles/articlesPrint.cfm?ID=227502 Accessed October 6, 2005.

Lewis JP. Fundamentals of Project Management. 2nd edition. New York: Amacom; 2002.

Lewis JP. The Project Manager's Pocket Survival Guide. New York: McGraw-Hill; 2003.

Littlejohns P, Wyatt J, Garvican L. Evaluating computerized health information systems: hard lessons still to be learnt. BMJ. 2003:326:860–863.

Loo, R. Project management: A core competency for professional nurse and nurse managers J Nurses Staff Dev. 2003;19(4):187–193.

Mantel S, Meredith J, Shafer S, Sutton M. Core Concepts: Project Management In Practice. Hoboken: John Wiley & Sons; 2005.

McCartney R. Leadership in nursing informatics. JOGNN. 2004;33: 371–380.

McGurkin T, Hart R, Millinghausen S. IT takes a care team. Nurs Manag. 2006; 37(3):18–31.

Mulcahy R. PMP Exam Prep: A Course in a Book Minneapolis: RMC Publications, 2002.

Pennypacker J, Cabanis-Brewin J. What Makes a Good Project Manager. Havertown, PA: Center for Business Practices; 2003.

Peters T. Leadership: Inspire, Liberate, Achieve. New York: Dorling Kindersley Limited;2005.

PM Forum. www.pmforum.org. Accessed April 3, 2007.

Poon E. Overcoming barriers to adopting and implementing computerized physician order entry systems in US hospitals. Health Affairs. 2004;3(4):184–190.

Portny SE. Project Management For Dummies. New York: Wiley Publishing; 2001.

Project Management Institute. http://www.pmi.org. Accessed March 25, 2007.

Project Management Institute's Healthcare Special Interest Group. http://www.pmihealthcare.org. Accessed April 17, 2007.

Rowen S. Project management vs. general management methodologies. PMI Baltimore Monthly. 2005;1:1–3.

Sargent S, Panico R. The structures of success: ten guidelines for sustainable program and project management. Insight. 2003;3(1):4–10.

Schwalbe K. Information Technology Project Management. Boston: Thompson Course Technology; 2006.

Scoble K, Russell G. Vision 2020, Part I: profile of the future nurse leader. JONA. 2003;33(6):324–330.

Smith P. A portrait of risk. PMI Network. 2003;17(4):45–48.

Staggers N, Gassert C, Curran C. A Delphi study to determine informatics competencies for nurses at four levels of practice. Nurs Res. 2002;51(6):383–390.

Tuckman. Forming, Storming, Norming, Performing Model. Business Ball. http://www.businessballs.com/tuckmanformingstormingnormingperforming.html Accessed September 8, 2005.

Upenieks V. Nurse leaders' perceptions of what compromises successful leadership in today's acute inpatient environment. Nurs Admin Q. 2003;27(2):140–152.

Urbanic C, Kemmeling D, Grunwald M. 2004. The project management office: putting it all together. HCT Project. Volume 2. July 17, 2004 http://www.hctproject.com/documents.asp?d_ID=1847# Accessed September 17, 2005.

Williams J, Murphy P. Better project manager and better patient outcomes. Nurs Manag. 2005;36(11): 41–47.

Wikipedia–Earned Value Management. http://en.wikipedia.org/wiki/Earned_value_management

Wikipedia–Project Management. http://en.wikipedia.org/wiki/Project_management

Wikipedia–Informatics. http://en.wikipedia.org/wiki/Informatics

Appendix

Table of Contents

Initiation Phase

Initiation Worksheet Template
Initiation Worksheet Sample
Charter Template A
Charter Template B
Charter Approval Form
Scope Template
Scope Sample: Small Project
Scope Sample: Large Project

Planning

Work Plan Template: Microsoft Excel
Risk Report Template
Risk Report Sample
Sample Communication Plan Grid

Execution and Control

Status Report Template
Meeting Minutes Template
Issue Log Template
Scope Change Request and Impact Analysis Template A
Scope Change Request and Impact Analysis Template B

Closing

Completion Document Template
Sample Completion Document
Lessons Learned Sample

Appendix

This appendix includes document templates and samples to provide an example of formats. Although it is important to include specific information in some of the documents mentioned in this book, the format can vary depending on your organization or project management methodology. These are meant to be examples only.

Initiation Phase

The Initiation phase begins with data gathering and ends with a charter document or a scope document. If the project manager finds it beneficial, a worksheet can be used to enter the data gathered that would be used for the final documents. This would provide a single place for this information to be documented before the charter and scope documents, but it is not necessary. If a worksheet is used, the information can be copied and pasted into the project charter or scope document.

Initiation Worksheet Template

XXX Organization PMO
Initiation Worksheet

This is a worksheet to help in the gathering of information in the Project Initiation Phase

Project Name:
Project Manager:

Business Need:

Goals:

Objectives:

Deliverables:

Constraints:

Assumptions:

Relevant Historical Information:

Resource Needs:

Initiation Worksheet Sample

XXX Organization PMO
Initiation Worksheet

This is a worksheet to help in the gathering of information in the Project Initiation Phase

Project Name: Project Management Office Creation
Project Manager: Susan M. Houston

Business Need:
  To improve success for projects run out of the XXX department by instituting standard and consistent methods for managing projects.

Goals:

- All projects managed from XXX department will utilize a standard methodology irrelevant to their size.
- 75% of all XXX department managed projects meet their Success Factors as identified in their scope document.
- Educate all XXX department staff to the new process of project management methodology.
- Educate current XXX department Project Managers in the new methodology required for managing projects assigned to them.

Objectives:

- Provide ongoing coaching and mentoring to all XXX department Project Managers.
- Provide education sessions to all XXX department Projects Managers related to the new methodology.
- Attend staff meetings to communicate new methodology to all staff.
- Place all templates and documents in a shared location for all staff to access.

Deliverables:

- Project Management Methodology Overview
- Project Document Templates and Examples
- PMO Education sessions

Constraints:

- Time available for this project
- Staffing resources for developing education materials
- Cost, if necessary, to purchase any software or contract personnel

Assumptions:

- Staff will accept the change if completed in small increments.
- Mentoring and additional education will be needed for some staff to fully understand and accept the new methodology.

Relevant Historical Information:

Staff in XXX department, and YYY organization in general, is resistant to change.

Resource Needs:

- Space for education sessions and meetings
- Dedicated project managers for each project
- Space for record keeping (library of project documentation for historical information)
- Training materials to hand out in education sessions

Charter Template A

XXX Organization PMO
Project Charter
Project Name

Prepared By: Date:

Project ID:
Project Name:
Business Group:

This Project Charter has been delivered, reviewed, and approved as shown below:

Stakeholder Name	Role	Dept./Area	Signatures	Date
	Project Sponsor			
	Project Sponsor			
	Project Manager			

Estimated start date:
Estimated finish date:

Business need and core benefits:
Why are we doing this project?

Background:
Indicate any background information that is pertinent to this project.

Objectives:
Identify the project's most critical objectives (preferably measurable).

Scope:
Identify what is in and out of scope for this project.

Project description and major deliverables:
What is this project supposed to accomplish? Indicate high-level deliverables or milestones critical to the project's success.

Critical measurements:
Identify important quantitative measurements that will be used to help evaluate the project's progress and success.

Success factors:
Identify those qualitative and quantitative elements (internal and external to the project) that will prove important to the project's success.

Stakeholders:

* Include all individuals who will play an active role in the decision-making in regard to the project.

Role	Name	Responsibility/title
Project Sponsor		
Project Manager		
Others		

Cost management:

* Include all project-related costs that may impact the project.

Estimated Costs	
Type of Cost	Amount

Project documentation:
The following project-related documents will be created and maintained throughout the implementation of the project.

Project Document	Owned By
Work plan	
Communication plan	
Risk Management plan	
Training plan	

Communication plan:

Meetings:

Reports:

Issue management:
Issues and key decisions will be tracked and managed using the PMO Issue Log.

Risk management:

Risk management involves proactive decision making and aggressive action taking.

Project closure:

Upon completion of the project, the Project Manager will communicate with all stakeholders and others who may have an interest in the status of the <project name >implementation.

Charter Template B

**XXX Organization PMO
Project Name
Project Charter**

Project
Sponsor:
Department:

Project Manager:

Start Date:

Approval Date:

Revision Date:

I. Introduction

A. Background
Provide background information about how the current situation evolved.

B. Current Environment / Situation
Describe how the current business process can be improved by implementing the proposed project.

C. Business Need
Describe the compelling business reasons why this project is important and why it should be approved and funded.

D. Stakeholders List
List the individuals playing key roles in the project.

E. Type of Project
Indicate the project type.

F. Project Types

☐ New Application   ☐ Data Management   ☐ Infrastructure
☐ HIPAA   ☐ New Process   ☐ JCAHO
☐ Interface   ☐ Upgrade   ☐ Other

II. Project Description

A. Objectives
Describe the objectives of this project.

B. Scope
Describe the boundaries of this project in terms of the high-level components to be delivered to the business to accomplish the objective stated above. Identify what is included in the scope of the project, and what is not included in the scope of the project.

1. Business units affected

2. Modules of the project

3. Functions within the project

4. Technology architecture–Infrastructure

5. Interfaces

6. Assumptions

7. Constraints

8. What is not in scope

9. What scope decisions have not been made

C. Alternative Solutions Considered
List alternative solutions considered to satisfy the business need.

D. Dependencies
Describe the business systems or technology that this project is dependent on for output, cross-functional teams, software, or applications that are dependent on the output of this project.

E. Risks
Describe the risks for the project.

III. Stakeholder Expectations and Measures of Success

Identify the expectations of the project stakeholders

A. Stakeholder Expectations

B. Business Performance Measures

C. Technical Performance Measures

D. Financial Performance Measures

IV. Estimated Project Cost

IS Capital Investment	Year 1	Year 2	Year 3
Hardware			
Software			
Interfaces			
Network			
Database			
Disaster Recovery			
Consulting for Contractors			
Capital Total			
Ongoing Incremental Operating IS Costs	**Year 1**	**Year 2**	**Year 3**
Annual Maintenance			
Annual Software License			
Network Expense			
Consulting for Contractors			
Training			
Staffing (FTE's)			
Disaster Recovery			
Support - Help Desk			
Configuration Management			
Operating Total			

V. Project Approach

A. Organization
Describe the different governing groups for the project (i.e., steering committee etc.).

B. Delivery Strategy
Describe the delivery strategy for components (i.e., "Big Bang" vs. "little steps) that will be delivered in each phase over the project's duration.

C. Milestones and Phases
Indicate the associated major project phases and associated milestone dates.

Milestone/Phase Name	Date:
Project Phase One:	
Milestone	
Milestone	
Milestone	
Project Phase Two:	
Milestone	
Milestone	
Milestone	

Charter Approval Form

Document Author:	Date:

List of Approvers:

Name	Department/Area Representing	Accepted Y/N

Action Item / Concerns / Issues	Assigned to	Due Date

Scope Template

XXX ORGANIZATION PMO
Project
SCOPE DOCUMENT

Mission Statement:

Project Objectives/Scope:
-

Project Justification
-

Leadership Roles:
    Project Sponsors:
    Project Manager:
    Project Resources:

Implementation Strategy:

Project Milestones:
    Milestone   *Estimated Completion Date*

Measures of Success:

Assumptions:

Constraints:

Project Sponsor   Date

Scope Sample: Small Project

This scope sample is for a small project and includes communication, risks, and training plans. A communication matrix should be included.

XXX ORGANIZATION PMO
Workstation Registration Website Development
SCOPE DOCUMENT

Mission Statement:

Provide a website that will allow end users, or technical staff, to enter workstation information to be registered in the EHR application, as well as a report for the project team to review the information entered.

Project Objectives:

- Create a website for end users and technical staff to provide information to the project team so they can register the workstations.
- The website will reside on the organization's intranet
- The website will utilize the organization's standard template for items such as color, fonts, etc.
- The website will provide directions for finding Workstation ID on PC or Mac computers
- There will be a report listing the workstations to be registered that will print daily and on demand

Project Justification

There are a variety of workstations available to the clinical staff. The hardware includes PCs and Macs. It is important to communicate detailed instructions to the technical support staff related to setting up workstations to access to the EHR application. It is necessary for each workstation to be entered into the EHR application to allow access. A mechanism for the end user and technical staff to provide the required information to the project team is also important.

Leadership Roles:

Project Sponsors: Gary Micheals
Project Manager: Sue Sapelak
Project Resources: Matthew Houston
                     Nicole Currie
                     Azrena Miller

Implementation Strategy:

The website will be developed and tested before any communication will go out. Communication related to the need to register the workstations will sent to all technical staff and the Desktop Support team.

Training Strategy:

There is no formal training required. Instructions will be in the communication going out and there will be a contact name/number for questions.

Communication Plan:

Communication to this staff would be done using multiple forums. The IT committee would be used for general information sharing. Dr Gary Hanson would present information to this group. Communication will also be done with regard to all Technical Staff using group email lists and listserves.

Risk Assessment:

Risk - There is a risk that not all workstations will be registered before the EHR go-live.

Mitigation – The help desk will be staffed with someone who can register the workstations if calls come in during and after go-live.

Project Milestones:

Milestone	Estimated Completion Date
Requirements Complete	March 16, 2006
Development Complete	April 13, 2006
Testing Complete	April 27, 2006
Communication out	April 29, 2006

Measures of Success:

- The application allows data entry and retains it in a database
- The data entered is available in a report that prints daily and on demand

Assumptions:

- All workstations accessing the EHR need to be registered
- Communication will be effective at notifying users to register their workstations

Constraints:

- Limited resources to develop website
- The website needs to be completed in time to register all workstations before the EHR go-live

_____   _____

Gary Michaels, Project Sponsor   Date

Scope Sample: Large Project

This scope sample is for a large project where communication, risks, and training plans are all separate documents.

XXX ORGANIZATION PMO
EHR Upgrade
SCOPE DOCUMENT

Mission Statement:

To upgrade the current EHR vs. 3.0 to a EHR vs. 4.0, which includes enhanced order entry, as well as multiple system-supplied enhancements.

Project Objectives:

- To upgrade the current 3.0 system to 4.0.
- To upgrade the current order entry to include pharmacy orders.
- There will not be any major changes or additions to the orders except pharmacy.
- To implement available features – features to be implemented will be added as addendum A once defined and approved.
- To update the training materials and user manuals related to changes made to the system during the upgrade.
- To provide training on new, or enhanced, features included in the upgrade.
- Training may be classroom, CBT, or written updates in the form of a newsletter depending on the scope of the changes.
- Upgrade interfaces as needed.
- The hardware and database migration strategy will be added as Addendum B once defined and approved.

Project Justification

- To improve order entry with improved pharmacy orders.
- To improve functionality of system with new features included in 4.0.

Leadership Roles:

Sponsor:	Gary Michaels
Project Manager:	Sue Sapelak
Project Leaders:	Nicole Houston, Order Configuration
	Matthew Currie, Technical
Project Resources:	Azrena Miller, Remainder
	Tom Pauls, Remainder and Orders
	Barb Armstrong, Orders
	Florence Palumbo, Reports
	Julia Jacubiak, Technical
	Frank James, Technical
	Julia Vincelli, Testing
	Toni Michelle, Interfaces
	Others may be defined later

Project Milestones:

Milestone	Estimated Completion Date
Access to 4.0 Development System	April 2006
Analysis and Build of Remainder Items	July 1, 2006
Analysis and Build of Orders	July 1, 2006
Access to 4.0 Test System	July 8. 2006
Testing Complete	August 15, 2006
Training Material Development Complete	August 25, 2006
Training Complete	September 26, 2006
Upgrade to 4.0	September 27, 2006

Measures of Success:

- All environments (dev, test, train, prod) upgraded to 4.0.
- Clinical staff using new orders.
- Interfaces modified as necessary and functioning correctly.

Assumptions:

- There is no need to change the hardware configuration for this upgrade, per the vendor.
- New features that require extensive analysis to determine extent of application will be implemented through Configuration Management after the upgrade.

New features that require extensive analysis related to plan for implementation and impact on processes will be implemented though Configuration Management after the upgrade.

Constraints:

- There are resource constraints for the new order build.
- There are hardware and process constraints related to process to upgrade environments to 4.0 while still supporting and providing Configuration Management releases for 3.0.

Gary Michaels, Project Sponsor   Date

Planning

Project planning includes the documentation, or use of standard plans, such as scope management plan, schedule management plan, resource management plan, and risk management plan. Although there should be standardization in how these are managed across projects, they are unique to the organization. Below are a few templates of documents the project manager will need to create outside of these plans.

Work Plan Template: Microsoft Excel

Often, a project work plan begins in Excel because the table can have blank fields and can easily be shared with other team members who may not have access to Microsoft Project. Once the initial work plan is finalized, it can be moved to Project. If the project is small, it could be kept in Excel.

Name	Effort	Duration	Start Date	Finish Date	Pred	Resource
Project Initiation						
Define Project Team						Sponsor
Define Scope						Sponsor / PM
Scope Approval						Sponsor
Define Communication Mgmt Plan						PM
Initial Project Plan						PM
Project Tasks						
High Level						
Middle Level						
Detailed Level						
High Level						
Middle Level						
Detailed Level						
High Level						
Middle Level						
Detailed Level						
Project Completion						
Project Completion Analysis						Sponsor / PM
Project Completion Document						PM
Project Completion Approval						Sponsor

Risk Report Template

Below is a template that can be used to identify and track risks and the mitigation strategies for a project.

XXX ORGANIZATION PMO
Project Risk Analysis

Purpose:

Objective/Scope:

Background:

Overall Assessment:

Documents used for the Report:

Document Change Record				
Rev #:	**Effective Date:**	**Purpose:**	**Approved by:**	**Signature/Date:**
1		Initial Submission		

Risks

1. *Risk:*

Recommendation:

2. *Risk:*

Recommendation:

3. *Risk:*

Recommendation:

4. *Risk:*

Recommendation:

5. *Risk:*

Recommendation:

Summary:

Risk Report Sample

XXX ORGANIZATION PMO
4.0 Upgrade RISK ANALYSIS

Purpose
The purpose of this report is to identify the risks and issues associated with upgrading the EHR version 3.0 to version 4.0.

Objective/Scope
The objective of this report is to assure all risks and issues are identified as early as possible so actions can be taken to mitigate these risks.

Background
The initial plan was to upgrade from version 3.0 to version 3.6. Planning initially occurred for the upgrade to 3.6 and the planning documents have since been reviewed and modified to reflect the decision to upgrade to 4.0.

Overall Assessment
There have been 2 risks surrounding the upgrade to 4.0. The risks are outlined in this document. Additional risks may be identified as the project progresses.

4.0 Upgrade Risks
A risk is defined as the potential for negative consequences to occur that have an impact to the project go-live schedule. Two risks were identified for the upgrade to 4.0 and are defined below. The risks will be reviewed by project manager. Actions taken to mitigate these risks will be documented and tracked to resolution.

6. Risk:
There may be a delay in procuring the hardware, which could affect the time allotted for hardware configuration. This could delay implementing the upgrade.
Mitigation Strategy:
The project manager should continue to monitor the process with hardware procurement and attempt to expedite the procurement and configuration process. To make efficient use of the time allotted for configuration, planning for configuration of the hardware should be developed as soon as the hardware is finalized so it can be implemented as soon as the hardware arrives.

2. Risk:
SCM 3.0 was an older solution believed to be more stable at the time than 4.0. There were still multiple critical issues after go-live for the implementation

of 3.0. SCM 4.0 is a new release and the vendor does not have any customers live on this version. If issues arise, the implementation could be delayed.

Mitigation Strategy:

Review all documentation from the vendor concerning known issues and determine the impact on the implementation. Log all implementation issues with the vendor and track their resolution. Additional implementation and testing time may need to be added or workarounds may need to be implemented for some of these issues.

Upgrade Risk Summary

The initial upgrade for the EHR was to upgrade from version 3.0 to version 3.6. The decision was made to upgrade to a more recent version, 4.0. The risks for the upgrade appear to be minimal at this point in the project. Additional risks may be identified as the project progresses. All risks should be tracked by the Project Manager to resolution.

Sample Communication Plan Grid

XXX ORGANIZATION PMO
Project
COMMUNICATION MANAGEMENT MATRIX

Who	What	When	How	Responsible
Board/ Steering Committee	Status	Monthly Meeting	Verbal Presentation	Project Sponsor
Administration	Status	Monthly Meeting	Verbal Presentation	Project Manager
Project Manager	Status	Regular Status Meetings	Verbal or Email	Project Team Members
End Users	Training Information	2 Months pre-live	E-mail, Flyers, Posters	Training Staff
End Users	Reminders of changes w/Upgrade	2 weeks pre-live blitz	E-mail, Flyers, Posters	Training Staff
Help Desk	Changes w/Upgrade impacting support	2 weeks pre-live	Discussion	Project Manager
Vendors	As tech assistance needed	As needed	Conf Calls	Project Manager
Project Team	Status, minutes, reports, work plan, etc	Weekly status meetings	Meetings and project documen- tation	Project Manager

Execution and Control

The execution and control phases occur concurrently and are the phases where the project manager ensures the planned activities are completed. All plans are executed, and the activities are controlled to follow each plan. The majority of communication occurs in the form of status reports, meeting minutes, and updates related to issues and changes.

Status Report Template

STATUS REPORT

TO: PROJECT DIRECTOR

FROM:

SUBJECT: STATUS REPORT

CC

DATE:

Actions/Tasks Completed:

Next Steps:
Late Tasks:

Task	Task Name	Start Date	Finish Date	% Complete

Tasks Scheduled to be completed this month

Task	Task Name	Start Date	Finish Date	% Complete

Tasks Scheduled to start next

Task ID	Task Name	Start Date	Finish Date	% Complete

Issues/Action Plans:

Logistics:

Meeting Minutes Template

[Meeting Name] Meeting Minutes
[Date]

I. Call to order

[Name of Meeting Facilitator] called to order the regular meeting of the [Organization/Committee Name] at [time of meeting] on [data of meeting] in [Location of Meeting].

II. Roll call

[Name of Organization Secretary] conducted a roll call. The following persons were present: [List of Attendees]

III. Approval of minutes from last meeting

[Name of Organization Secretary] read the minutes from the last meeting. The minutes were approved as read.

IV. Open issues

 a) [Open issue/summary of discussion]
 b) [Open issue/summary of discussion]
 c) [Open issue/summary of discussion]

V. New business

 a) [New business/summary of discussion]
 b) [New business/summary of discussion]
 c) [New business/summary of discussion]

VI. Adjournment
[Name of Meeting Facilitator] adjourned the meeting at [time meeting ended].
Minutes submitted by: [Name]
Minutes approved by: [Name]

Issue Log Template

Project Title
ISSUE LOG
Last Updated:

ISSUE #	DATE OPENED	DATE DUE	ISSUE	RESPONSIBLE INDIVIDUAL	STATUS
1					
2					
3					
4					
5					
6					
7					
8					
9					
10					
11					
12					

Scope Change Request and Impact Analysis Template A

Change Request Form

Directions: Please complete this form when requesting modifications to any part of the system that is not within the scope of the project and/or identified on the project work plan. Provide supporting documentation when possible and return to an SMS representative. This request will be reviewed by the project management team for a recommended action.

Request Opened By	Department/Title	Phone Number	Fax Number

Brief Description of Change Request

Impact to LIVE Comment/Explanation		YES	NO
Can the system go LIVE without the change request?			
Impact to LIVE date.			
Will the Change Request require post-LIVE maintenance/support?			

Detailed Reason for Request: Include implications to operational practices (Attach pages if needed)

Impact Analysis

Time Estimates - what is the initial estimate of work effort?	☐ Minimal (1–3 hours) ☐ Average (4–8 hours) ☐ Extensive (8 + hours)
Staffing Resources – will this change require changes in staffing levels and skill sets?	
Budget Allocations/Cost – will this change require additional professional services?	
Testing Phase – will this change impact the Testing Phase. Explain.	
Training Phase – will this change impact the Training Phase. Explain.	
Elimination of other tasks – what tasks could be delayed to post live ?	
Have other alternatives been considered, if so please list.	

Additional pages attached?   YES   NO

Application Consultant Review

Applications Involved:

Analysts who reviewed request: Date

Comments:

Project Management Review

Course of Action   Date

Deny			* If accepted, persons responsible for request or PSR number.
Post-Live			
Accepted*			

Comments:

Reviewed By:

VENDOR Project Manager   Date

ABC Hospital Project Manager   Date

Steering Committee (if applicable)   Date

Scope Change Request and Impact Analysis Template B

Project
Scope Change Request

Project Name:	Project Code #:
Project Sponsor:	Submitted By:
	Date Requested:

Type:

Description:

Desired Change and Impact of Not Making the Change:

Disposition: Approved   Denied   Deferred

Approval:

_____   _____
Sponsor   Date

_____   _____
Leader   Date

Closing

At the end of the project, the project completion document is completed. If the project is small, the lessons learned could be included in the completion document. Larger projects usually have lengthier lessons learned documents and it is better to have them in a separate document

Completion Document Template

XXX ORGANIZATION PMO
Project
COMPLETION DOCUMENT
date

Scope Statement:

Project Sponsor:

Project Leader:

Project Manager:

Project Team:

Measures of Success/Expected Outcomes:

Constraints:

Expected Timeframe:

Major Project Milestones:

_____	_____
Project Sponsor	Date
_____	_____
Project Manager	Date

Sample Completion Document

XXX ORGANIZATION PMO
Workstation Registration Website Development
PROJECT COMPLETION ANALYSIS DOCUMENT

Mission Statement:
Provide a website that will allow end users, or technical staff, to enter workstation information to be registered in the EHR application as well as a report for the project team to review the information entered.

Project Sponsor: Gary Michaels
Project Manager: Sue Sapelak

Project Scope/Objectives:

- Create a website for end users and technical staff to provide information to the project team so they can register the workstations. *Done*
- The website will reside on the organization's intranet. *Done*
- The website will utilize the organization's standard template for items such as color, fonts, etc. *Done*
- The website will provide directions for finding Workstation ID on PC or Mac computers. *Done, although it did not include directions for Mac OS9*
- There will be a report listing the workstations to be registered that will print daily and on demand. *Done*

Measures of Success/Expected Outcomes:

- The application allows data entry and retains it in a database. *Met*
- The data entered is available in a report that prints daily and on demand. *Met*

Implementation Strategy:
The website will be developed and tested before any communication will go out. Communication related to the need to register the workstations will sent to all technical staff and DNA's Desktop Support team. *This strategy was followed without modification.*

Risk Impact:
Risk - There is a risk that not all workstations will be registered before the EHR go-live.
Mitigation – The help desk will be staffed with someone who can register the workstations if calls come in during go-live. *This risk did not impact this project because it relates to after the CRIS go-live, which occurs in the future. This risk will be added to the CRIS Risk list.*

Constraints:

- Limited resources to develop website. *There was only one development resource available on the project. He was able to spend sufficient amount of time working on his tasks and the timeline was not impacted.*
- The website needs to be completed in time to register all workstations before the EHR live. *Because the EHR project was delayed, this constraint did not impact the project.*

Major Project Milestones:

Milestone	Est Completion Date	Actual Completion Date
Requirements Complete	March 16, 2006	March 16, 2006
Development Complete	April 13, 2006	April 15, 2006
Testing Complete	April 27, 2006	April 27, 2006
Communication out	April 29, 2006	April 29, 2006

The development took longer than expected, but because the testing went smoothly, there was not a delay in the rollout of the website. The communication did go out on time, but follow-up communication continued for approximately a week to ensure complete communication.

Sponsor Comments:

_____   _____

Gary Michaels, Project Sponsor   Date

Lessons Learned Sample

XXX ORGANIZATION PMO
4.0 Upgrade Lessons Learned

Purpose

The purpose of the EHR Implementation Lessons Learned Report is to present key lessons learned by the system implementation team during the 4.0 upgrade from the procurement of the application through go-live. The objective of the document is to provide information gathered during the implementation so future projects might benefit from its successes and learn from its areas for improvement, and thereby improve the implementation process as a whole.

Project Management and Communication
Project Successes

- o The early clarification of roles and responsibilities for each project team member and reaching agreement on project expectations were important organizational tasks.
- o The Steering Committee, Project Sponsors, along with the senior management, actively supported and monitored the program's status, including the weekly schedule revisions and risks. This is a critical component to managing program scope, budget, and timelines, and future projects should develop similar oversight structures.

Areas for Improvement

- o Technical resources need to be involved in the relevant program areas early in the project planning. The technical limitations of a system can have a significant impact on the maintenance of that system and those issues should be known and owned much earlier in the process.

Design and Build
Project Successes

- o Regular meetings on various subtasks of the project, such as Interfaces, Testing, and Infrastructure, helped to ensure identification, communication, and resolution of key issues identified within those areas.
- o Valid Interface Requirement Definitions Document was maintained throughout the development and testing phases.

Areas for Improvement

- o Start design and development of reports earlier, and involve the user departments throughout the process.
- o Design documents should be completed before the build phase.

System Testing
Project Successes

- o The operational parallel tests conducted within the hospital were well planned and staffed to test inpatient and outpatient processes using the new version in parallel to the old. There was invaluable feedback obtained regarding issues with the system as well as with planned processes. The issues were evaluated and categorized into "fix by live," "training," "Frequently Asked Questions (FAQs)," and "future needs." All fix by live issues were resolved before live, and the FAQs were also published before live.
- o The UAT scripts and scenarios involved real life scenarios, which helped identify issues that were not identified in other areas of testing. Some scenarios were reused from Integration Testing and some new scripts were written based on feedback from users for areas not previously tested.

Areas for Improvement

- o Allow Time For Retesting. Due to the delays in Build, some functionality was not thoroughly tested before Go-Live.
- o All development should be completed before the start of Testing.

Training
Project Successes

- o The process followed for dissemination of user passwords worked effectively for both the users and the system administrators. Users were not provided their passwords until they had successfully completed training, which ensured only qualified users were given access to the system.
- o The Training Team adapted well to issues that arose, such as changes in schedule, room size issues, changes to training materials, etc. This adaptability allowed the team to accommodate special training needs to assure all staff received the proper training.

Areas for Improvement

- o None identified.

Activation/Deployment Planning
Project Successes

- o A detailed activation checklist included all tasks required for the 3 days before go-live. This was developed with the project team involvement and was detailed down to 5-minute tasks for the night of the upgrade. This was very beneficial in keeping staff on track with what was being done. A large version of this checklist was posted in various locations with staff identified to check off the tasks as they were completed so everyone knew the progress or the impact of delays.

o The identification and training of dedicated staff to support activation was crucial to the success of go-live. This training included Disaster Recovery and Fail-Over exercises.

Areas for Improvement

o The Call Center would have initially been more effective at go-live if they had been provided end user training and access to the application in the production environment.

Lessons Learned Summary

The most successful area of the project was the testing phase. The testing phase was the strongest because the plans for each phase of testing were very comprehensive and the test team adapted the plans seamlessly to the dynamic testing conditions.

Index

A

Actual cost (AC), 60
Administrators/knowledge management
    coordinators, 12
American National Standards
    Institute/Electronic Industry
    Association, 60
Archiving, of project records, 5, 68
Assumptions
    definition of, 19
    effect of constraints on, 27
    as project charter component, 19
    in project management office
        development, 80
    in risk identification, 28

B

Bibliography, 95–97
Budget coordinators, 10–11
Budgets, 27, 57–59
    components of, 59
    contingency, 64, 75
    cost of work performed, 60
    final verification of, 64
    overruns on, 64, 93
    strategic, 92
    of system implementation projects, 74–75
Business analysts, 6, 12
Business needs analysis, 16–17

C

Change control process, 92
Charters, of projects, 4, 15, 16, 91
    applications of, 91
    approval form for, 110
    current state, 18
    definition of, 18–19
    final review of, 32
    for system implementation projects, 72
    for system selection projects, 70
    templates of, 81, 104–110

Closing phase, 1, 5, 6, 81, 84
    completion document templates for, 128–130
    components of
        celebration, 68
        documentation of lessons learned, 65–66
        end of project, 68
        formal acceptance, 66–68
        verification, 63–65
    definition of, 63, 128
    lessons-learned sample of, 131–133
    of training program development projects, 88
Communication, 92
    during execution and control phases,
        40–43, 120
    within functional organizations, 22
    with stakeholders and sponsors, 29, 48, 54,
        92–93
Communication plans, 16, 29–30, 41, 76, 91
    sample grid of, 120
Completion document, 63, 66–68, 81, 88, 128
    templates for, 81, 128–130
Constraints
    definition of, 19
    impacts on, 27
    as project charter component, 19
    in project management office
        development, 80
    in risk identification, 28
    in system implementation projects, 75
    triple, 2–3
Constructive cost model, 28
Contingency budgets, 64, 75
Contingency planning, 51
Contract officers, 12
Control phase, 51–61, 81, 92
    assessment of project performance in,
        54–55, 58
    budget management in, 58–59
    corrective action in, 57–58
    definition of, 120
    earned value management (EVM) in, 60–61
    key benefit of, 51

reconfirmation of project plans in, 52–54
of research projects, 90
of system implementation projects, 73–75
Corrective action, 57–58
Cost
  as constraint on projects, 2–3
  final analysis of, 5
  of human resources, 27
  parametric modeling, 28
  Top-down estimates, 28
Cost estimates, 16, 27–28, 71, 92
Cost performance index (CPI), 60–61
Cost variance (CV), 60, 61
Current state, as project charter component, 18
Current state documentation, 17–18
Current state model, 83

D
Deliverables
  high-level, 18
  in project management office
    development, 80
Director/managers, of project management
  offices, 6, 7–8
Directors, of project management offices, 6,
  7–8

E
Earned value management (EVM), 60–61
Electronic health records (EHRs), 31–33
End user groups, 17–18
Estimate at completion (EAC), 61
Execution phase, 1, 4–5, 35–49, 81, 92
  components of
    communication, 40–43
    issue management, 45–46
    norming phase, 46–47
    performing phase, 48
    project resource management, 36–37
    project team formation, 37–47
    quality control, 48
    storming phase, 37, 43–44
  definition of, 35–36, 120
  of research projects, 90
  of system implementation projects, 73–75
  templates used in, 121, 124–128
Executive committees, 29–30

F
Flow diagrams, of current state documentation,
  17–18
Functional managers, 22–23
Future state, 17, 18, 83

G
Goals
  definition of, 17, 91
  organizational, 17
  as project charter component, 18
  in project management office
    development, 80
  shared, 92

H
High-level estimates, 18
Historical information, 16
  effect on project time, 21–22
  lessons learned documents as, 65
  in project management office development,
    79, 80
  in research projects, 89
  in risk identification, 28
Human resources
  cost of, 27
  estimates for, 18
  management, 54

I
"Icebreaker" exercises, 38–40
Impact analysis templates, 124–128
Information distribution, as project manager's
  role, 4–5
Information systems, purchasing of, 92
Information technology projects, failure of, 93
Initiation phase, 1, 3–4, 5, 15–20,
    91–92
  components of
    current state documentation, 17–18
    historical information, 16
    needs analysis, 16–17
    project charter, 18–19
    project goal definition, 17
    project objectives definition, 17
    project scope documents, 19–20
    project selection, 15–16
    risk assessment, 19
    roles and responsibilities, 20
  definition of, 15
  of research projects, 89
  of system implementation projects, 72
  templates and forms used in
    charter approval form, 110
    charter template, 104–110
    scope sample, 112–115
    scope template, 111
    worksheets, 100

worksheet sample, 102–103
worksheet template, 101
Interdisciplinary care model, 83–84, 85–86
Issue logs, 45–46
  templates of, 123
Issue management, 45–46

K
Kickoff meetings, 32–33, 37

L
Leadership skills, of project managers, 43–44,
  46, 48, 55–57, 77, 92
Lessons learned, from projects
  as completion document component, 81
  from interdisciplinary care projects, 85–86
  from research projects, 90
  sample of, 131–133
Lessons learned documents, 65–66
Lessons learned meetings, 65

M
Meeting minutes, 120
  templates of, 81, 122
Milestones, of projects, 67
Mind mapping, 25

N
Needs analysis/assessment, 16–17,
  18, 69–70
Network diagrams, 26
Networking, among project managers, 57
Nurse managers, 91

O
Objectives
  conflict between, 17
  definition of, 17, 91
  organizational, 17
  planning of. *See* Planning phase
  as project charter component, 18
  in project management office
    development, 80
  shared, 92
Organizations, types of, 22–23

P
Parametric modeling, of cost estimation, 28
Percentage complete (%Comp.), 61
Performance, components of, 4
Physician Computer Order Entry, 69, 72

Plan(s)
  approval of, 32
  definition of, 32
  final review of, 32–33
  reconfirmation/reevaluation of, 52–54, 56
  for system selection projects, 69–70
Planned value (PV), 60
Planning, definition of, 21
Planning phase, 1, 4, 5, 21–33, 81, 91–92
  components of
    communication, 29–30
    contingency planning, 51
    cost estimates, 16, 27–28, 92
    kickoff meetings, 32–33, 37
    risk management, 28
    time estimates, 16, 26, 27
    work (project) plan, 23–27, 84, 85,
      89–90, 91
  definition of, 116
  for end-use training, 32
  goals of, 81
  for hardware deployment, 31–32
  importance of, 21
  of quality management plans, 31
  of research projects, 89
  of resource planning, 31
  risk report sample for, 118–119
  risk report templates of, 117
  sample communication plan grid of, 120
  of schedule management, 31
  of scope management, 30–31
  of system implementation projects, 73–74
  of system selection projects, 70–71
  work plan templates of, 116
Processes, 1–2
  transition to, 83
Procurement audits, 63
Project(s)
  authorization of, 18
  definition of, 1, 2, 35
  differentiated from processes, 1–2
  failure of, 51, 52
  milestones, 67
  modifications of, 3
  system implementation, 72–75, 76
  system selection, 69–71
Project Management Institute, 1, 80
Project management office (PMO), 6–13, 92
  definition and functions of, 6
  development of, 79–80
    initiation worksheet for, 81–82
    initiation worksheet in, 81–82
    tasks in, 82
  documentation of project progress in, 76

goals of, 80
roles in, 6–13
of systems implementation projects, 72–75
of systems selection projects, 69–71
Project management process, 1–13, 92–93. *See also* Closing phase; Controlling Phase; Execution phase; Initiation phase; Planning phase
applications of
in healthcare informatics, 69–77
in healthcare management, 79–90
definition of, 1, 91
Project managers, 6, 8–9
accountability of, 3
authority of, 3, 20
identification of, 15–16
leadership skills of, 43–44, 46, 48, 55–57, 77, 92
in matrix organizations, 22
mistakes made by, 56
as project team leaders, 23
responsibilities of, 20, 57
training and mentoring of, 81, 82
Project planners/schedulers, 11
Project teams, 22–23
development of, 37–48
ground rules for, 38
"icebreaker" exercises for, 38–40
norming phase, 37, 46–47
performing phase, 37, 48
storming phase, 37, 43–44
leaders of, 6, 10
performance assessment of, 54–55, 58

Q
Quality assurance process, 57–58, 92
Quality control, 48
Quality management plans, 31

R
RACI model, of project process documentation, 76
Research projects, 89–90
Resource management plans, 116
Resource needs, in project management office development, 80
Resource planning, 31
Resources, 2. *See also* Human resources
analysis/estimation of, 18, 81
management of, 31, 36–37, 116
requests for, 58

Risk(s)
analysis/evaluation of, 16, 19, 28
definition of, 19
effect of constraints on, 27
identification of, 19, 28
management of, 28, 73, 91, 116
mitigation of, 16, 19, 28, 86
Risk management plans, 28, 91, 116

S
Schedule(s), 3
adherence to *versus* modification of, 51
status reports on, 40–43
Schedule control, 57–58
Schedule management plans, 31, 116
Schedule performance index (SPI), 61
Schedule variance (SV), 60, 61
Scope
changes to, 47, 53, 66–67
request template of, 124–128
control of, 46–47
creep, 30
as constraint on projects, 2–3
definition of, 18, 46, 91
final evaluation/documentation of, 5, 66–67
management plans – 4, 30, 31, 81, 116
of research projects, 89
sample of, 112–115
of system selection projects, 71
templates of, 81, 111
Scope documents, 4, 19–20, 63, 91
applications of, 91
final review of, 32
management, 57–58
of research projects, 90
of training programs, 87–88
Software implementation projects, human resource estimates for, 18
Sponsors, 4
acceptance of project outcomes by, 63, 66–68
approval of project charters by, 91
approval of scope documents by, 91
communication plans for, 29
definition of, 20
multiple, 72
project methodology information for, 81–82
roles and responsibilities of, 20
Stakeholders
communication plans for, 29
communication with, 29, 48, 54, 92–93
definition of, 3, 20
identification of, 3
information needs of, 58
project methodology information for, 81–82

reconfirmation of project plans by, 52–54
roles and responsibilities of, 20
senior, as project sponsors, 4
status reports for, 41
of system selection projects, 70, 71
Status meetings, 41, 53
Status reports, 36–37, 40–43, 44,
    48–49, 76, 120
in control phase, 58
sample of, 74
sample template of, 43, 44
stoplight format of, 41, 42
in system implementation projects, 73, 74
templates of, 43, 44, 81, 121
Steering committees, 29–30
Supervisors, role in resource management,
    36–37
System implementation projects, 72–75, 76
Systems analysts, 13
System selection projects, 69–71

T
Tasks, high-level, 24, 25, 70
Time (duration), of projects
as constraint, 2–3
effect of historical information on, 21–22
estimates of, 16, 26, 27
final analysis of, 5

To-complete performance index (TCPI), 61
Top-down cost estimates, 28
Total cost of ownership (TCO), 59
Training plans, 81
Training programs, 84, 86–88
Triple constraint, 2–3

U
User acceptance testing (UAT), 63

V
Validation, of projects, 81, 88

W
Work breakdown structure. See Work
    (project) plans
Work (project) plans, 23–26, 91
Analogy approach, 25
Appendix, 99–133
Bottom-up approach, 25
definition of, 92
of interdisciplinary care projects, 84, 85
project time estimation component of, 27
of research projects, 89–90
sample of, 118–119
templates of, 116
Work schedules. See Schedules